# ENDURANCE EXERCISE and ADIPOSE TISSUE

# CRC Series in Exercise Physiology

*Series Editor*
Ira Wolinsky

## Published Titles

CONCEPTS in FITNESS PROGRAMMING
*Robert G. McMurray*

EXERCISE and DISEASE MANAGEMENT
*Brian C. Leutholtz and Ignacio Ripoll*

PHYSIQUE, FITNESS, and PERFORMANCE
*Thomas Battinelli*

MUSCULOSKELETAL FATIGUE
AND STRESS FRACTURES
*David B. Burr and Chuck Milgrom*

# ENDURANCE EXERCISE and ADIPOSE TISSUE

*Edited by*

**Barbara Nicklas**

# CRC PRESS

Boca Raton   London   New York   Washington, D.C.

Cover art is used with permission from Mohamed-Ali, V., Pinkey, J.H., and Coppack, S.W., Adipose tissue as an endocrine and paracrine organ, *Int. J. Obesity*, 22, 1146, 1998.

## Library of Congress Cataloging-in-Publication Data

Endurance exercise and adipose tissue / edited by Barbara Nicklas.
    p. ; cm.
Includes bibliographical references and index.
ISBN 0-8493-0460-1 (alk. paper)
    1. Adipose tissues—Metabolism. 2. Exercise—Physiological effect. I. Nicklas, Barbara.
[DNLM: 1. Adipose Tissue—metabolism. 2. Exercise—physiology. QS 532.5.A3 E56 2001]
QP88.15 .E535 2001
612.3'97—dc21                                    2001043359

### Visit the CRC Press Web site at www.crcpress.com

# Preface

Adipose tissue, once considered inert connective tissue, is an essential storage site for key substrates that are used as sources of energy. Adipocytes have numerous metabolic functions, the most important of which are the hydrolysis (lipolysis), uptake, and storage of triacylglycerol. The regulation of adipocyte lipid metabolism during periods of excess energy expenditure is critical for the maintenance of fuel homeostasis. For example, adipocytes adapt to acute and long-term increases in physical activity by enhancing their capacity to mobilize and replenish lipid, which is used for energy by exercising muscle. Furthermore, in recent years, cellular and molecular biologists have advanced the concept that adipocytes are not solely a cellular storage location for excess fuel. Rather, adipose tissue is an active secretory organ that synthesizes and releases a number of bioactive proteins, which influence energy and substrate metabolism throughout the body via endocrine, paracrine, and/or autocrine actions.

The exercise-induced adaptations in muscle metabolism are widely recognized and thoroughly studied across several disciplines. Yet, despite the important role of adipose tissue in providing fuel for exercise and its newly recognized role as an endocrine organ, exercise-induced adaptations in adipose tissue are far less familiar. This book is solely dedicated to providing exercise physiologists, nutritionists, medical professionals, and basic scientists with concise and current information regarding the effects of endurance exercise on adipose tissue metabolism, mass, and distribution. Each chapter is written by leading scientific researchers with specific expertise and first-hand knowledge of the subject of their chapters. Where appropriate, for each metabolic function, the necessary basic science is explained first, followed by a comprehensive review and interpretation of the scientific literature pertaining to the effects of endurance exercise on that metabolic function.

This book is designed to give the reader timely, current insight into the exercise-induced metabolic adaptations in adipose tissue metabolism and their clinical significance. The first few chapters focus on the effects of endurance exercise on the primary metabolic functions of adipocytes. Included are the effects of both a single exercise bout and endurance exercise training on adipose tissue lipolysis, lipoprotein lipase, and glucose uptake and insulin responsiveness. One chapter also summarizes the effects of endurance exercise on the endocrine/paracrine properties of adipose tissue, a newly developing area of research. The book concludes with three chapters that examine the evolving research on the effects of endurance exercise on adipose tissue mass and body fat distribution. Although these topics have been historically presented in the context of the effects of exercise on body composition or obesity, the chapters written for this book highlight the unique capacity of endurance exercise to modify adipocyte size and the amount and location of adipose tissue in children and adults. The hope is that these chapters will provide an applied approach to the basic information presented on exercise and adipocyte metabolism and that this book will serve as a text and reference source for scientists and clinicians alike.

The preparation of this book required the hard work and dedication of each of the contributing authors and their assistants. They deserve gratitude and thanks for their willingness to contribute their expertise to this volume in such a creative, timely, and professional manner.

# The Editor

**Barbara J. Nicklas, Ph.D.,** is associate professor of Internal Medicine in the Section on Gerontology and Geriatric Medicine at Wake Forest University School of Medicine, Winston-Salem, NC. Dr. Nicklas received her Ph.D. in Exercise Physiology from the University of Maryland at College Park. As a National Institutes of Health (NIH)-sponsored postdoctoral research fellow at the University of Maryland at Baltimore, Dr. Nicklas conducted research investigating the effects of weight loss and exercise on *in vitro* adipocyte lipolysis, lipoprotein lipase activity, lipid metabolism, body fat distribution, and body composition in obese, postmenopausal women. From 1996 to 2001, she was assistant professor in the Division of Gerontology at the University of Maryland, Baltimore, where she continued to study the effects of exercise on adipose tissue metabolism and distribution in older women.

Dr. Nicklas' broad research focus is on studying the genetic and cellular mechanisms responsible for the adverse health effects of weight gain, inactivity, and accumulation of abdominal adipose tissue in older men and women. In the past, her research has been supported by grants from the NIH, the American Heart Association, and the Veterans Administration. Her contributions to knowledge in this area are demonstrated by her publication record, which includes more than 40 journal articles, a book chapter, and two review papers, as well as more than 35 published abstracts. She also regularly presents research findings at national meetings.

Dr. Nicklas is a member of five professional organizations: the American College of Sports Medicine, the American Diabetes Association, the American Physiological Society, the North American Association for the Study of Obesity, and the Gerontological Society of America. She serves as a peer reviewer on a regular basis for several journals, including the *American Journal of Physiology, Journal of Applied Physiology, Journal of Clinical Endocrinology and Metabolism, International Journal of Obesity, Obesity Research,* and the *American Journal of Clinical Nutrition.* In addition, Dr. Nicklas has served as an advisor to the NIH, as a member of two NIH Special Emphasis Review Panels, as a member of the Subcommittee B Study Section for the National Institute of Diabetes and Digestive and Kidney Diseases, and as a consultant in the National Institutes of Aging extramural Geriatrics Program office.

# Contributors

**Dora M. Berman, Ph.D.**
Division of Gerontology
University of Maryland, and
Baltimore Geriatric Research
  Education and Clinical Center
Virginia/Maryland Health Care
  System
Baltimore, Maryland

**Matthew S. Hickey, Ph.D.**
Departments of Health and Exercise
  Science, Physiology, and Food
  Science and Human Nutrition
Colorado State University
Fort Collins, Colorado

**Jeffrey F. Horowitz, Ph.D.**
Division of Kinesiology
University of Michigan
Ann Arbor, Michigan

**Richard G. Israel, Ed.D.**
Department of Health and Exercise
  Science
Colorado State University
Fort Collins, Colorado

**Ian Janssen, Ph.D.**
School of Physical and Health
  Education
Queen's University
Kingston, Ontario, Canada

**Samuel Klein, M.D.**
Department of Internal Medicine
Center for Human Nutrition
Washington University School
  of Medicine
St. Louis, Missouri

**Barbara J. Nicklas, Ph.D.**
Gerontology and Geriatric
  Medicine
Wake Forest University
Winston-Salem, North Carolina

**Robert Ross, Ph.D.**
School of Physical and Health
  Education
Department of Medicine
Division of Endocrinology and
  Metabolism
Queen's University
Kingston, Ontario, Canada

**Alice S. Ryan, Ph.D.**
Division of Gerontology
University of Maryland School
  of Medicine
Baltimore, Maryland

**Richard L. Seip, Ph.D.**
Hartford Hospital
Hartford, Connecticut

**Bente Stallknecht, M.D., Ph.D.**
Copenhagen Muscle Research
  Centre
Department of Medical Physiology
University of Copenhagen
Copenhagen, Denmark

**Margarita S. Treuth, Ph.D.**
Center for Human Nutrition
School of Public Health
Johns Hopkins University
Baltimore, Maryland

# Contents

*chapter one*

# Exercise and adipose tissue *lipolysis* in vitro

*Barbara J. Nicklas and Dora M. Berman*

## Contents

## 1.1  Introduction

One of the most important metabolic functions of adipose tissue is the hydrolysis (lipolysis) of triacylglycerol (TG) and the subsequent release of non-esterified fatty acids (NEFAs) and glycerol. Because NEFAs are a significant fuel source for oxidation by working muscles, the hormonal regulation of this process during periods of excess energy expenditure is critical for the maintenance of fuel homeostasis, especially during long-term bouts of endurance exercise. Circulating levels of catecholamines and insulin, the main hormonal regulators of lipolysis, are altered during exercise to stimulate adipocyte lipolysis and provide additional NEFAs. Moreover, evidence

0-8493-0460-1/02/$0.00+$1.50
© 2002 by CRC Press LLC

suggests that adipocytes adapt to acute and chronic increases in energy expenditure by enhancing their sensitivity to these hormonal regulators and increasing their capacity to mobilize NEFAs for generation of adenosine triphosphate (ATP) by exercising muscle.

This chapter summarizes the effects of endurance exercise on the lipolytic capacity and sensitivity of adipose tissue measured *in vitro*. Although results obtained using *in vitro* techniques may not directly reflect actual NEFA release from intact adipose tissue,[1] this method is very useful for studying adipocyte lipolysis under controlled conditions. Thus, the cellular adaptations that lead to exercise-induced changes in lipolysis can be delineated. The information in this chapter focuses on studies performed on humans for whom the levels of adipocyte lipolysis were measured before and after both a single exercise bout and endurance exercise training. A summary of what is known regarding the cellular mechanisms for adaptations in adipocyte lipolysis in response to endurance exercise is provided, as is information on the effects of gender, obesity status, and adipose tissue region.

## 1.2   Regulation of lipolysis in human adipose tissue

### 1.2.1   The lipolytic cascade

Dole[2] showed that one of the principal metabolic functions of adipose tissue is to hydrolyze stored TG into NEFAs and glycerol. Today, the complex steps leading to this reaction in the adipocyte are well known (see Figure 1.1). Lipolysis is regulated through a chain of events that involve hormone binding and the coupling of the hormone–receptor complex to the membrane-bound enzyme, adenylate cyclase. Lipolytic hormones bind to their receptors and activate the stimulatory guanine ($G_s$) nucleotide protein, while antilipolytic hormones bind to their receptors and activate the inhibitory guanine ($G_i$) nucleotide protein. The balance between these opposing pathways determines the magnitude of cyclic adenosine monophosphate (cAMP) production by adenylate cyclase. The concentration of cAMP controls the activity of cAMP-dependent protein kinase, which ultimately controls the phosphorylation and activation state of hormone-sensitive lipase (HSL), which is the rate-limiting enzyme that catalyzes the hydrolysis of TG into diglycerides and monoglycerides.[3] Ultimately, monoglycerides are hydrolyzed into glycerol and NEFA by monoacylglycerol lipase, which is not regulated by hormones.[4] Thus, the regulation of HSL activity is the most important factor in the mobilization of lipids from adipocytes.

The NEFAs hydrolyzed from TG are either re-esterified by the adipocyte or released to the plasma, where they bind to albumin and are transported to other tissues for oxidation and/or TG synthesis. The glycerol released during lipolysis is not reutilized by the adipocyte but is transported to the liver or kidney, where it is converted to glucose via glycerol kinase and other gluconeogenic enzymes.[5] Cyclic AMP is degraded to 5′-AMP via a phosphodiesterase-catalyzed reaction. Intracellular phosphatases dephosphorylate and

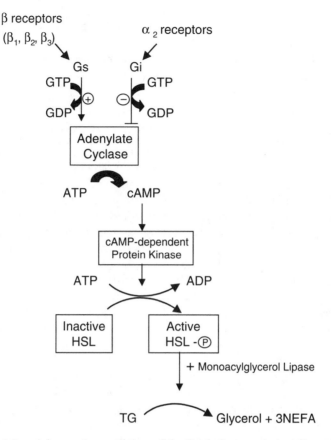

***Figure 1.1***    Adrenergic regulation of the lipolytic cascade in adipocytes.

inactivate protein kinase and HSL. Through this series of reactions, NEFAs, stored as TG in adipocytes, are made readily available as a source of energy substrate for other body tissues.

## 1.2.2   Hormonal regulation

The release of NEFAs from adipose tissue is regulated by hormones acting on the adipocyte. In humans, insulin and the catecholamines are the most physiologically important hormones regulating adipocyte lipolysis. Insulin is a potent antilipolytic hormone, the effects of which are mediated through receptor and postreceptor mechanisms.[6,7] Insulin stimulates phosphodiesterase subtype 3, thus reducing cAMP levels, which is the second messenger in the lipolytic cascade.[8] Insulin also promotes the inactivation of HSL through activation of protein phosphatase,[9] and, in addition, it stimulates the internalization of β-adrenergic receptors, which mediate catecholamine-stimulated lipolysis.[10] Norepinephrine secreted from nerve endings in adipose tissue or epinephrine and norepinephrine released from the adrenal medulla are the main stimulatory hormones of lipolysis.[11] Catecholamines exert a dual effect in humans, either stimulating lipolysis via β-adrenergic receptors ($\beta_1$, $\beta_2$, $\beta_3$)[12] or inhibiting lipolysis via $\alpha_2$-adrenergic receptors.[13] Under normal conditions, the lipolytic β effect dominates, but the balance in the density and affinity of these receptors can change so that catecholamines have a net inhibitory effect on lipolysis.[11]

### 1.2.3  *Measurement of adipocyte lipolysis* in vitro

Subcutaneous adipose tissue metabolism is measured *in vitro* in samples of adipose tissue obtained by a needle biopsy.[14] The biopsy can be conducted in any subcutaneous adipose tissue site, although the lower abdomen and upper gluteal/femoral regions are most frequently used. After the adipose tissue is removed, experiments are performed on whole pieces of the tissue or on isolated cells obtained by treating the tissue with collagenase to separate the adipocytes.[15] Adipocyte lipolytic sensitivity and maximal responsiveness to stimulatory or inhibitory agonists are measured *in vitro* using a double radioisotope technique[16] or by measuring the concentration of the end products, NEFA and glycerol, as indices of the lipolytic rate. Because NEFAs can be esterified into new TG for reutilization by adipocytes, the release of glycerol is a more accurate index of lipolysis. Glycerol is not reutilized by human adipocytes due to their lack of glycerol kinase, the enzyme necessary for metabolizing glycerol.[17]

To determine the lipolytic response to catecholamines, it is common to perform dose-response curves for the lipolytic response to norepinephrine and epinephrine, which result from both $\alpha_2$- and β-adrenoceptor stimulation. In general, the lipolytic response to norepinephrine has a sigmoidal shape, while the response to epinephrine has a biphasic shape with antilipolysis at low concentrations (preferential recruitment of $\alpha_2$-adrenoceptors), and a net lipolytic response at higher concentrations (approx. $\leq 10^{-6}$ $M$) (preferential recruitment of β-adrenoceptor).[18] Both sensitivity, estimated as $EC_{50}$ (which is the concentration of agonist necessary for half-maximal stimulation of lipolysis), and responsiveness can be obtained from the dose-response curve. Only a fraction of the available $\alpha_2$- and β-adrenoceptors need to be occupied in order to produce a maximal effect in isolated adipocytes. Thus, changes in sensitivity may reflect alterations in hormone action at or near the receptor level (i.e., receptor numbers), while changes in responsiveness are usually linked to changes in hormone action at postreceptor steps, such as coupling efficiency between the receptors and $G_s/G_i$ proteins, activities of phosphodiesterase, and hormone-sensitive lipase.[19] Because responsiveness to catecholamines results from stimulation of both $\alpha_2$- and β-adrenoceptors, selective adrenergic agonists are commonly used to discriminate between the antagonistic effects of the two receptors.

Adenosine is generated endogenously as an end product of cAMP degradation by phosphodiesterase, and, after binding to its own receptor, it inhibits adenylate cyclase and lipolysis by activating $G_i$ proteins.[20]

Addition of adenosine deaminase (ADA) removes adenosine from the medium, resulting in increased lipolysis. Thus, it is common to evaluate the inhibitory action of selective $\alpha_2$-agonists, as well as insulin, on basal lipolysis levels, which have been raised by addition of ADA. Selective adrenergic agonists to discriminate between $\alpha_2$- and $\beta$-adrenoceptors include clonidine and UK-14304 (selective $\alpha_2$-agonists), isoproterenol (non-selective $\beta$-agonist), terbutaline and procaterol (selective $\beta_2$-agonists), and dobutamine (selective $\beta_1$-agonist).[21,22]

Some agents act at well-defined steps beyond receptor stimulation, such as forskolin (adenylate cyclase activator), dibutyryl-cyclic AMP (a phosphodiesterase-resistant cAMP analog that stimulates the protein kinase/HSL complex), and enprofylline and theophylline (phosphodiesterase inhibitors). This battery of pharmacological agents is generally used to characterize the step at which different interventions such as exercise training and caloric restriction act to modify the *in vitro* lipolytic response of isolated adipocytes. The interventions may affect *in vitro* lipolysis by altering the functional balance between $\alpha_2$- and $\beta$-adrenoceptors and/or at postreceptor sites. Nevertheless, extrapolation of *in vitro* results to *in vivo* situations has to be done cautiously because several endocrine and other factors (e.g., adenosine, prostaglandins, NEFA, blood flow) affect basal lipolysis *in vivo*.

## 1.3   Effects of endurance exercise on adipocyte lipolysis

### 1.3.1   Effects of a single exercise bout

The oxidation of lipids is important for meeting the body's excess energy demands during exercise, especially exercise of a low to moderate intensity.[23] Up to 90% of the total energy expended during this type of exercise may be supplied by oxidation of NEFAs.[24] The NEFAs used for this enhanced fat oxidation is derived from circulating TG-rich lipoproteins in plasma, intramuscular TG stores, and circulating albumin-bound NEFAs mobilized from adipose tissue. Adipose tissue is the most important source of NEFA during prolonged bouts of endurance exercise.[25] Consequently, physiological changes occur during exercise to enhance the lipid mobilization from adipose tissue. Specifically, sympathetic nervous system activity increases, resulting in elevated catecholamine levels, which stimulate adipocyte lipolysis.[26] In addition, insulin concentration decreases during a prolonged exercise bout, reducing the inhibitory effects of insulin on lipolysis. These hormonal changes raise circulating levels of NEFAs and glycerol during continuous exercise, indicative of an increase in NEFA mobilization from adipose tissue. During higher intensity exercise, the accumulation of lactate inhibits HSL activity and reduces lipid mobilization from adipose tissue, allowing muscles to utilize glycogen as an energy source.[27] Furthermore, *in vitro* studies examining the effects of acute exercise on adipose tissue lipolysis suggest these hormonal changes are complemented by changes in adipocytes themselves to further enhance NEFA mobilization during exercise.

Studies using *in vitro* techniques show that adipocytes become more responsive to catecholamine stimulation during endurance exercise (see Table 1.1). This phenomenon was first documented in rat[28,29] and later in human[30-32] adipocytes taken immediately after an exercise bout. In one study, maximal catecholamine-stimulated lipolysis in abdominal adipocytes increased by 23% in young, lean males after 90 minutes of cycling exercise at 88% of maximal heart rate, but basal lipolysis was unchanged.[30] Similar results were seen in gluteal fat cells from a combined group of young men and women after 30 minutes of cycling exercise at 67% of maximal aerobic capacity ($VO_2$max).[31] The latter study demonstrated that the cellular mechanism responsible for the exercise-induced increase in catecholamine-stimulated lipolysis was an increase in β-adrenergic receptor responsiveness rather than changes in either β- or $α_2$-adrenergic receptor sensitivity. Moreover, radioligand-binding experiments showed that the increase in β-adrenergic receptor responsiveness was not due to a change in the availability of β-adrenergic receptor binding sites. These findings indicate that the exercise-induced increase in catecholamine-stimulated lipolysis is due to enhancement of a step in the β-adrenergic pathway that is distal to receptor binding.

Not all studies demonstrate an increase in catecholamine-stimulated lipolysis with acute endurance exercise;[32,33] however, discrepant results among studies are most likely due to differences in the gender of the subjects or the site of the adipose tissue sampled. In an attempt to clarify the effects of gender and fat location on adipocyte changes in lipolysis induced by acute exercise, both abdominal and gluteal adipocyte lipolysis were examined in separate groups of men and women before and after 30 minutes of cycling exercise at 67% of $VO_2$max.[32] Similar to previous findings, exercise did not affect basal lipolysis in either abdominal or gluteal adipose tissue in men or women. In abdominal adipocytes, exercise did not change catecholamine-stimulated lipolysis in either the men or women. However, in gluteal adipocytes, exercise increased catecholamine-stimulated lipolysis in men but

*Table 1.1*   Summary of the Effects of Acute Endurance Exercise on Basal and Catecholamine-Stimulated Abdominal and Gluteal Adipocyte Lipolysis in Men and Women

| Study | Abdominal | | Gluteal | |
|---|---|---|---|---|
| | Basal | Stimulated | Basal | Stimulated |
| Savard et al.[30] (men) | — | ↑ | NA | NA |
| Wahrenberg et al.[31] (men and women) | NA | NA | — | ↑ |
| Crampes et al.[33] (women) | — | — | NA | NA |
| Wahrenberg et al.[32] (men) | — | — | — | ↑ |
| (women) | — | — | — | — |

*Note:*  Dashed lines indicate no change; NA indicates not applicable (not studied); ↑ indicates an increase.

not in women. Furthermore, exercise increased postreceptor-stimulated lipolysis by 30% in gluteal adipocytes in men but not in women. This lack of an increase in catecholamine-stimulated lipolysis after exercise in women was due to greater $\alpha_2$-adrenergic antilipolytic responsiveness in gluteal cells, as the $\beta$-adrenergic responsiveness was equally enhanced in both men and women. The lack of an increase in lipolytic responsiveness in abdominal adipocytes in men contradicts an earlier finding,[30] but the discrepancy may be due to differences in the length of the exercise stimulus (e.g., 90 vs. 30 minutes).

In summary, *in vitro* adipose tissue lipolysis is increased during and immediately after exercise due to changes in concentrations of regulatory hormones, as well as changes in the lipolytic capacity of the adipocyte itself (Table 1.1). However, this effect varies depending on the length of the exercise session, the location of adipose tissue studied, and the gender of the subjects. This effect may be more pronounced in gluteal compared to abdominal adipocytes, as an increase in lipolysis of abdominal adipose tissue was only seen after a longer exercise bout. The mechanism for this exercise-induced increase in catecholamine-stimulated lipolysis is not due to changes in adrenergic receptors. It is due to enhancement of a step in the $\beta$-adrenergic receptor pathway that is distal to receptor binding. The biological function of this increase in adipocyte lipolysis following an acute exercise bout may be to provide a continuous flow of NEFAs to be used as substrates for energy production by working muscles during prolonged exercise of low to moderate intensity.

## 1.3.2   Effects of exercise training

Physiological adaptations occur after a period of endurance exercise training to improve the transport of oxygen to muscle and to change the relative resting substrate oxidation rate toward a greater reliance on lipids for energy production.[34, 35] In muscle, this shift in substrate utilization results from an increased capacity for lipid oxidation and a greater hydrolysis of intramuscular TG. In addition, results from both cross-sectional and exercise training studies show there is a concurrent training-induced adaptation in adipose tissue to increase its capacity for NEFA mobilization.[33,36-41]

### 1.3.2.1   Cross-sectional studies

Parizkova and Stankova[42] were the first to report a greater lipolytic responsiveness to catecholamine stimulation in adipocytes of exercise-trained rats. Subsequently, studies in humans confirmed and extended this finding. When abdominal adipocytes from male endurance athletes and sedentary men are compared, the basal rate of lipolysis is similar, but lipolytic responsiveness and sensitivity to catecholamine stimulation are greater in athletes due to an increase in the efficiency of the $\beta$-adrenergic pathway.[36,37] Similar results are seen in abdominal adipocytes of competitive female athletes compared with sedentary women, except that the increase in catecholamine-stimulated lipolysis in the athletes is due to a greater $\beta$-adrenergic stimulation, as well as a reduction in $\alpha_2$-adrenergic inhibition of lipolysis.[33,37,40,41] Three of these studies[33,40,41] showed that dibutyryl cAMP (dcAMP)-stimulated lipolysis (an analog of cAMP that diffuses into the cell and activates protein kinase) is also higher in women athletes. This indicates that the greater responsiveness of the $\beta$-adrenergic pathway in abdominal adipocytes of trained athletes may result from an adaptation that is distal to adenalyte cyclase in the lipolytic cascade.

### 1.3.2.2 Longitudinal studies

Only a few longitudinal studies in humans have examined the effects of endurance exercise training on adipose tissue lipolysis. In one study, 20 weeks of exercise increased $VO_2$max by 29% in young, lean men and by 33% in young, lean women. It did not change the basal rate of abdominal adipocyte lipolysis; however, catecholamine-stimulated lipolysis increased by 66% in the men and 46% in the women.[39] In a similar study, 20 weeks of endurance exercise training increased abdominal adipocyte catecholamine-stimulated lipolysis in men but not in women.[43] These results demonstrate a gender difference in the magnitude of the response of adipose tissue lipolysis to exercise training. Another study showed that basal and catecholamine-stimulated lipolysis were significantly higher in marathon runners and men who had exercise-trained for 20 weeks than in sedentary men.[44] However, lipolytic responsiveness did not differ between the recently trained men and the marathon runners, indicating that the lipolytic capacity of adipose tissue does not progressively increase with the duration of exercise training. It is also likely that genetic factors influence the effects of exercise training on adipose tissue lipolysis, as the magnitude of the increase in catecholamine-stimulated lipolysis after exercise training was more similar within than between pairs of twins.[45]

These previous longitudinal, as well as cross-sectional, studies were all performed in healthy, non-obese subjects. Because adipocyte responsiveness and sensitivity to catecholamines and/or insulin may be altered in obese individuals,[46-48] it is of interest to determine whether the effects of endurance exercise on adipocyte lipolysis are similar in obese subjects. For this purpose, adipocyte sensitivity to catecholamines and insulin was studied before and after 3 months of cycle ergometer exercise training in obese males (body mass index = $37 \pm 1$ kg/m$^2$).[38] Results showed that basal lipolysis and HSL activity decreased with training, but no changes were observed in lipolysis stimulated with postreceptor agonists. On the other hand, the lipolytic effects of epinephrine and $\beta$-agonists increased, and the antilipolytic effects of $\alpha_2$-adrenergic receptor agonists and insulin decreased. These combined effects suggest that, similar to non-obese subjects, exercise training enhances the capacity for NEFA breakdown and release in abdominal subcutaneous adipocytes of obese men.

We performed an exercise training study in obese, older women to determine whether the addition of endurance exercise to a 6-month dietary-induced weight loss program would prevent the decline in adipocyte lipolytic responsiveness seen with caloric restriction alone.[49] Basal, adrenergic-receptor-stimulated, and postreceptor-stimulated lipolysis in both abdominal and gluteal subcutaneous adipocytes decreased by 20 to 70% in women who underwent only caloric restriction, but did not change in women who underwent a combination of endurance exercise and caloric restriction. This suggests that the metabolic adaptations of adipose tissue to endurance exercise training could counteract the decrease in lipolysis associated with dietary-induced weight loss.

Although prior research consistently shows that lipolytic capacity and sensitivity of abdominal adipocytes are enhanced with endurance exercise, only one of these studies investigated whether or not regional differences exist in this response to exercise training. Mauriege et al.[40] showed that lipolytic responsiveness and sensitivity to catecholamine stimulation are greater in abdominal adipose tissue of female athletes compared with sedentary women, but they observed no differences in gluteal adipocyte lipolysis between trained and sedentary women. Thus, although further studies are needed, the ability of endurance exercise training to increase the capacity for NEFA release may be limited to the abdominal fat depot.

Cumulatively, these findings suggest that abdominal adipocyte responsiveness and sensitivity to catecholamine stimulation are enhanced with endurance exercise training, mostly due to changes in the stimulatory β-adrenergic receptor pathway of the lipolytic cascade. This lipolytic adaptation occurs within 20 weeks of training and occurs in both lean and obese men, but it may be greater in men than women. Because previous longitudinal studies examined the effects of endurance exercise training in abdominal adipose tissue only, it is unknown whether or not regional differences in the response of adipose tissue to endurance exercise training exist.

## 1.3.3  Cellular mechanisms

The results of the studies mentioned previously suggest that endurance exercise training enhances the capacity of adipose tissue to mobilize NEFAs; however, the cellular mechanisms for this adaptation are unknown, especially in humans. Results of one study in rats suggest that differences in adipocyte size between trained and untrained rats could account for the increased adipocyte lipolysis after exercise training.[50] Likewise, one of the cross-sectional studies in women found that the differences in lipolysis between endurance-trained athletes and sedentary women were the result of differences in adipocyte size. However, other results dispute this idea, as increased adipocyte lipolysis did not relate to variations in adipocyte size after exercise training,[39,51] nor did expressing lipolytic activity per cell size affect the magnitude of the increase in lipolysis observed between trained and sedentary men and women in two other studies.[37,41] Thus, a discrepancy currently exists regarding whether or not exercise training has an effect, per se, on adipocyte lipolysis that is independent of differences in adipocyte size.

This exercise-training-induced adaptation in adipocytes could potentially occur at any or all of the biochemical steps in the lipolytic cascade (see
Figure 1.1). Because each of these steps has been studied more thoroughly
in rats than humans, data from both models are reviewed here. First, lipolysis
may be enhanced with exercise training by an increase in receptor number
or binding affinity; however, in rats, exercise training had no effect on hormone binding to fat cell membranes taken from epididymal fat pads.[50,52] This
finding suggests that the lipolytic capacity of rat adipocytes increases with
endurance exercise training through a step distal to receptor binding. At
present, no studies in humans have examined the effects of endurance exercise on adrenergic receptor number or binding affinity.

Endurance exercise training also may influence the adenylate cyclase
activation/cAMP formation step of lipolysis; however, results of rat studies
that investigated this are conflicting. One study found that adenylate cyclase
activity was lower,[53] while others found it was higher,[52,54] in exercise-trained
compared with untrained rats. The latter two studies suggest that, in rats,
exercise training could enhance lipolysis by increasing receptor-cyclase coupling.[52,54] These conflicting results may be due to differences in the gender
of the rats studied or to methodological differences in the measurement of
adenylate cyclase activity. Studies examining the effects of exercise training
on hormone-stimulated cAMP formation show that, at every concentration
of lipolytic agonist, trained rats accumulate less cAMP than untrained littermates.[55,56] Additionally, cAMP accumulation was lower after fat cell stimulation with isoproteronol in trained rats even though their lipolytic rates
were elevated compared to their littermates.[55,56] The finding of an elevated
level of phosphodiesterase, the enzyme responsible for the breakdown of
cAMP, in both of these studies suggests that exercise training enhances
lipolysis by some mechanism other than increasing cAMP levels, possibly
by increasing the activity of protein kinase or HSL. Likewise, in humans,
adipocytes from exercise-trained subjects show a greater lipolytic response
to cAMP stimulation than adipocytes from untrained subjects.[37,40,41] This
finding also points to an adaptation in the protein kinase/HSL steps of the
lipolytic cascade with endurance exercise training.

In a study of the final steps of the lipolytic process (i.e., protein kinase
and HSL), endurance exercise training did not change protein kinase activity
of adipose tissue from female rats.[53] However, in another study, exercise
training reduced the activity of protein kinase, suggesting a decreased capacity to activate HSL.[57] Similarly, HSL activity was lower in exercise-trained
compared with control rats[56] and higher in rats after 13 weeks of treadmill
running.[58] In humans, the only available data regarding the effects of endurance exercise training on protein kinase or HSL activity or expression in
adipocytes show that HSL activity decreases with 12 weeks of endurance
exercise training in obese men.[38]

It is also important to note a study that reported elevated activities of
mitochondrial enzymes in white adipose tissue of swim-trained rats.[59]
Because lipolysis requires ATP, this enhanced ability to synthesize ATP may

contribute to the increase in adipocyte lipolysis with exercise training. Thus, to date, no definitive mechanism explains the enhanced rate of adipocyte lipolysis after endurance exercise training in rats or humans. The most feasible mechanism for greater epinephrine-stimulated lipolysis following exercise training is based on the data showing a training-induced increase in lipolysis after cAMP stimulation. This suggests that exercise training alters adipocyte lipolytic responsiveness at a step that is distal to adenylate cyclase, probably by increasing expression and/or phosphorylation of HSL.

## 1.4   Summary

The physiological purpose of the exercise-induced adaptations in adipose tissue lipolysis is to increase its capacity to release lipid substrates during exercise. Both adipocyte responsiveness and sensitivity to catecholamine stimulation increase during a single bout of exercise and after a period of endurance exercise training. Additional research is needed to determine whether or not the interaction of other factors such as age, gender, genotype, body composition, body fat distribution, and dietary habits alter the response of adipocyte lipolysis to endurance exercise. It is also necessary to clarify whether exercise-induced changes in lipolysis differ between adipose tissue sites and if these regional adaptations in adipocyte lipolytic capacity provide a mechanism for alterations in body fat distribution with exercise training. Elucidation of these details will provide information regarding the most effective exercise prescription for reducing abdominal obesity and cardiovascular disease (CVD) risk factors in overweight, sedentary populations.

## References

1. Lillioja, S., Foley, J., Bogardus, C., Mott, D., and Howard, B., Free fatty acid metabolism and obesity in man: *in vivo* and *in vitro* comparisons, *Metabolism*, 35, 505, 1986.
2. Dole, V., A relation between non-esterified fatty acids in plasma and the metabolism of glucose, *J. Clin. Invest.*, 35, 150, 1956.
3. Fain, J. and Garcia-Sainz, J., Adrenergic regulation of adipocyte metabolism, *J. Lipid Res.*, 24, 945, 1983.
4. Large, V. and Arner, P., Regulation of lipolysis in humans. Pathophysiological modulation in obesity, diabetes, and hyperlipidaemia, *Diabetes and Metabolism*, 24, 409, 1998.
5. Fain, J., Hormonal regulation of lipid mobilization from adipose tissue, in *Biochemical Actions of Hormones*, Academic Press, New York, 1980.
6. Bjorntorp, P. and Ostman, J., Human adipose tissue dynamics and regulation, *Adv. Metab. Disord.*, 5, 277, 1971.
7. Lonnroth, P. and Smith, U., The antilipolytic effect of insulin in human adipocytes requires activation of the phophodiesterase, *Biochem. Biophys. Res. Commun.*, 141, 1157, 1986.
8. Gegerman, E., Belfrage, P., and Manganiello, V., Structure and regulation of cGMP-inhibited phosphodiesterase (PDE3), *J. Biol. Chem.*, 272, 6823, 1997.

9. Stralfors, P., Olsson, H., and Belfrage, P., Insulin-induced dephosphorylation of hormone-sensitive lipase, *Eur. J. Biochem.*, 182, 379, 1989.
10. Engfeldt, P., Hellmer, J., Wahrenberg, H., and Arner, P., Effects of insulin on adrenoceptor binding and the rate of catecholamine-induced lipolysis in isolated human fat cells, *J. Biol. Chem.*, 263, 15553, 1988.
11. Arner, P., Control of lipolysis and its relevance to development of obesity in man, *Diabetes/Metab. Rev.*, 4, 507, 1988.
12. Lafontan, M., Differential recruitment and differential regulation by physiological amines of fat cell $\beta_1$, $\beta_2$ and $\beta_3$-adrenergic receptors expressed in native fat cells and in transfected cell lines, *Cell. Signal.*, 6, 363, 1994.
13. Galitzky, J., Mauriege, P., Berlan, M., and Lafontan, M., Human fat cell alpha-2 adrenoceptors, I. Functional exploration and pharmacological definition with selected alpha-2 agonists and antagonists, *J. Pharmacol. Exp. Ther.*, 249, 583, 1989.
14. Hirsch, J., Farquhar, J., Ahrens, E., Peterson, M., and Stoffel, W., Studies of adipose tissue in man: a microtechnic for sampling and analysis, *Am. J. Clin. Nutr.*, 8, , 1960.
15. Rodbell, M., Metabolism of isolated fat cells, I. Effects of hormones on glucose metabolism and lipolysis, *J. Biol. Chem.*, 239, 375, 1964.
16. Leibel, R., Hirsch, J., Berry, E., and Gruen, R., Radioisotopic method for the measurement of lipolysis in small samples of human adipose tissue, *J. Lipid Res.*, 25, 49, 1984.
17. Steinberg, D., Vaughan, M., and Margolis, S., Studies of triglyceride biosynthesis in homogenates of adipose tissue, *J. Biol. Chem.*, 236, 1631, 1961.
18. Mauriege, P., Prud'homme, D., Lemieux, S., Tremblay, A., and Despres, J., Regional differences in adipose tissue lipolysis from lean and obese women: existence of postreceptor alterations, *Am. J. Physiol. (Endocrinol. Metab.)*, 269(32), E341, 1995.
19. Arner, P., Hellmer, J., Wennlund, A., Ostman, J., and Engfeldt, P., Adrenoceptor occupancy in isolated human fat cells and its relationship with lipolysis rate, *Eur. J. Pharmacol.*, 146, 45, 1988.
20. Kather, H., Bieger, W., Michel, G., Aktories, K., and Jakobs, K., Human fat cell lipolysis is primarily regulated by inhibitory modulators acting through distinct mechanisms, *J. Clin. Invest.*, 76, 1559, 1985.
21. Mauriege, P., Imbeault, D., Langin, D., Lacaille, M., Almeras, N., and Tremblay, A., Regional and gender variations in adipose tissue lipolysis in response to weight loss, *J. Lipid Res.*, 40, 1559, 1999.
22. Reynisdottir, S., Ellerfeldt, K., Wahrenberg, H., Lithell, H., and Arner, P., Multiple lipolysis defects in the insulin resistance (metabolic) syndrome, *J. Clin. Invest.*, 93, 2590, 1994.
23. Saltin, B. and Astrand, P., Free fatty acids and exercise, *Am. J. Clin. Nutr.*, 57(suppl.), 752S, 1993.
24. Paul, P., Effects of long-lasting physical exercise and training on lipid metabolism, in *Metabolic Adaptation to Prolonged Physical Exercise*, H.H. Poortsmans, Ed., Birkhauser Verlag, Basel, 1975, p. 186.
25. Bulow, J. and Madsen, J., Regulation of fatty acid mobilization from adipose tissue during exercise, *Scand. J. Sports Sci.*, 8, 19, 1986.
26. Galbo, H., *Hormonal and Metabolic Adaptations to Exercise*, Georg Thieme Verlag, Stuttgart, 1983.

27. Boyd, A., Giamber, S., Mager, M., and Lebovitz, H., Lactate inhibition of lipolysis in exercising man, *Metabolism*, 23, 531, 1974.
28. Barakat, H., Kerr, D., Tapscott, E., and Dohm, G., Changes in plasma lipids and lipolytic activity during recovery from exercise of untrained rats, *Proc. Soc. Exp. Biol. Med.*, 166, 162, 1981.
29. Savard, R., Smith, L., Palmer, J., and Greenwood, M., Site-specific effects of acute exercise on muscle and adipose tissue metabolism in sedentary female rats, *Physiol. Behav.*, 43, 65, 1988.
30. Savard, R., Despres, J., Marcotte, M., Theriault, G., Tremblay, A., and Bouchard, C., Acute effects of endurance exercise on human adipose tissue metabolism, *Metabolism*, 36, 480, 1987.
31. Wahrenberg, H., Engfeldt, P., Bolinder, J., and Arner, P., Acute adaptation in adrenergic control of lipolysis during physical exercise in humans, *Am. J. Physiol. (Endrocinol. Metab.)*, 253, E383, 1987.
32. Wahrenberg, H., Bolinder, J., and Arner, P., Adrenergic regulation of lipolysis in human fat cells during exercise, *Eur. J. Clin. Invest.*, 21, 534, 1991.
33. Crampes, F., Beauville, M., Riviere, D., Garriques, M., and Lafontan, M., Lack of desensitization of catecholamine-induced lipolysis in fat cells from trained and sedentary women after physical exercise, *J. Clin. Endocrinol. Metab.*, 67, 1011, 1988.
34. Henriksson, J., Training-induced adaptation of skeletal muscle and metabolism during submaximal exercise, *J. Physiol.*, 270, 661, 1977.
35. Holloszy, J. and Coyle, E., Adaptations of skeletal muscle to endurance exercise and their metabolic consequences, *J. Appl. Physiol.: Respirat. Environ. Exercise Physiol.*, 56, 831, 1984.
36. Crampes, F., Beauville, M., Riviere, D., and Garrigues, M., Effect of physical training in humans on the response of isolated fat cells to epinephrine, *J. Appl. Physiol.*, 61, 25, 1986.
37. Crampes, F., Riviere, D., Beauville, M., Marceron, M., and Garrigues, M., Lipolytic response of adipocytes to epinephrine in sedentary and exercise-trained subjects: sex-related differences, *Eur. J. Appl. Physiol.*, 59, 249, 1989.
38. De Glisezinski, I., Crampes, F., Harant, I., Berlan, M., Hejnova, J., Langin, D., Riviere, D., and Stich, V., Endurance training changes in lipolytic responsiveness of obese adipose tissue, *Am. J. Physiol.*, 275, E951, 1998.
39. Despres, J., Bouchard, C., Savard, R., Tremblay, A., Marcotte, M., and Theriault, G., The effect of a 20-week endurance training program on adipose-tissue morphology and lipolysis in men and women, *Metabolism*, 33, 235, 1984.
40. Mauriege, P., Prud'homme, D., Marcotte, M., Yoshioka, M., Tremblay, A., and Bouchard, C., Regional differences in adipose tissue metabolism between sedentary and endurance-trained women, *Am. J. Physiol.*, 273, E497, 1997.
41. Riviere, D., Crampes, F., Beauville, M., and Garrigues, M., Lipolytic response of fat cells to catecholamines in sedentary and exercise-trained women, *J. Appl. Physiol.*, 66, 330, 1989.
42. Parizkova, J. and Stankova, L., Influence of physical activity on a treadmill on the metabolism of adipose tissue in rats, *Br. J. Nutr.*, 18, 325, 1964.
43. Despres, J., Bouchard, C., Savard, R., Tremblay, A., Marcotte, M., and Theriault, G., Effects of exercise training and detraining on fat cell lipolysis in men and women, *Eur. J. Appl. Physiol.*, 53, 25, 1984.

44. Despres, J., Bouchard, C., Savard, R., Tremblay, A., Marcotte, M., and Theriault, G., Level of physical fitness and adipocyte lipolysis in humans, *J. Appl. Physiol.: Respirat. Environ. Exercise Physiol.*, 56, 1157, 1984.

45. Despres, J., Bouchard, C., Savard, R., Prud'homme, D., Bukowiecki, L., and Theriault, G., Adaptive changes to training in adipose tissue lipolysis are genotype dependent, *Int. J. Obesity*, 8, 87, 1984.

46. Mauriege, P., Despres, J., Prud'homme, D., Pouliot, M., Marcotte, M., Tremblay, A., and Bouchard, C., Regional variation in adipose tissue lipolysis in lean and obese men, *J. Lipid Res.*, 32, 1625, 1991.

47. Reynisdottir, S., Wahrenberg, H., Carlstrom, K., Rossner, S., and Arner, P., Catecholamine resistance in fat cells of women with upper-body obesity due to decreased expression of $\beta_2$-adrenoceptors, *Diabetologia*, 37, 428, 1994.

48. Johnson, J., Fried, S., Pi-Sunyer, F., and Albu, J., Impaired insulin action in subcutaneous adipocytes from women with visceral obesity, *Am., J. Physiol. Endocrinol. Metab.*, 280, E40, 2001.

49. Nicklas, B., Rogus, E., and Goldberg, A., Exercise blunts declines in lipolysis and fat oxidation after dietary-induced weight loss in obese older women, *Am. J. Physiol.*, 273, E149, 1997.

50. Bukowiecki, L., Lupien, J., Follea, N., Paradis, A., Richard, D., and LeBlanc, J., Mechanism of enhanced lipolysis in adipose tissue of exercise-trained rats, *Am. J. Physiol. (Endocrinol. Metab. 2)*, 239, E422, 1980.

51. Owens, J., Fuller, E., Nutter, D., and DiGirolama, M., Influence of moderate exercise on adipocyte metabolism and hormonal responsiveness., *J. Appl. Physiol.: Respirat. Environ. Exercise Physiol.*, 43, 425, 1977.

52. Williams, R. and Bishop, T., Enhanced receptor-cyclase coupling and augmented catecholamine-stimulated lipolysis in exercising rats, *Am., J. Physiol. (Endocrinol. Metab.)*, 243, E345, 1982.

53. Shepherd, R., Sembrowich, W., Green, H., and Gollnick, P., Effect of physical training on control mechanisms of lipolysis in rat fat cell ghosts, *J. Appl. Physiol.*, 42, 884, 1977.

54. Izawa, T., Komabayashi, T., Tsuboi, M., Koshimizu, E., and Suda, K., Augmentation of catecholamine-stimulated [³H] GDP release in adipocyte membranes from exercise-trained rats, *Jpn. J. Physiol.*, 36, 1039, 1986.

55. Askew, E., Hecker, A., Coppes, V., and Stifel, F., Cyclic AMP metabolism in adipose tissue of exercise-trained rats, *J. Lipid Res.*, 19, 729, 1978.

56. Shepherd, R., Noble, E., Klug, G., and Gollnick, P., Lipolysis and cAMP accumulation in adipocytes in response to physical training, *J. Appl. Physiol.: Respirat. Environ. Exercise Physiol.*, 50, 143, 1981.

57. Oscai, L., Caruso, R., Wergeles, A., and Palmer, W., Exercise and the cAMP system in rat adipose tissue, I. Lipid mobilization, *J. Appl. Physiol.*, 50, 250, 1981.

58. Askew, E., Huston, R., Plopper, C., and Hecker, A., Adipose tissue cellularity and lipolysis, *J. Clin. Invest.*, 56, 521, 1975.

59. Stallnecht, B., Vinten, J., Ploug, T., and Galbo, H., Increased activities of mitochondrial enzymes in white adipose tissue in trained rats, *Am., J. Physiol. (Endocrinol. Metab.)*, 261, E410, 1991.

*chapter two*

# Endurance exercise and adipose tissue lipolysis in vivo

*Jeffrey F. Horowitz and Samuel Klein*

## Contents

0-8493-0460-1/02/$0.00+$1.50
© 2002 by CRC Press LLC

## 2.1   Introduction

Adipose tissue is the largest fuel reserve in the human body. Even lean adults usually have more than 100,000 kcal of potential energy stored as triglycerides in adipose tissue, which is approximately 50-fold more than the amount stored as glycogen in skeletal muscle and liver. The use of adipose tissue as a fuel during exercise requires the coordinated regulation of triglyceride lipolysis, adipose tissue blood flow (ATBF), and skeletal muscle blood flow to enhance the delivery of released fatty acids from adipose tissue to working muscles. Adipose tissue triglycerides are an important source of fuel during exercise. The increase in lipolytic rate that occurs during exercise facilitates delivery of fatty acids from adipose tissue to skeletal muscle for oxidation. This increase in fatty acid availability to muscle requires the integration of neural, hormonal, and circulatory events. This chapter reviews the factors that regulate lipolysis of adipose tissue triglycerides, the methods used to measure whole-body and regional lipolytic activity *in vivo*, and the effect of dietary intake, obesity, aging, and endurance training on the mobilization and use of endogenous triglycerides during exercise.

## 2.2   Lipolytic regulation of adipose tissue triglycerides

Lipolysis of adipose tissue triglycerides is stimulated through a cascade of signals resulting in the phosphorylation and activation of hormone-sensitive lipase (HSL), which is the enzyme that catalyzes triglyceride hydrolysis. Once phosphorylated, HSL translocates from the cytosol of the adipocyte to the surface of the lipid droplet within the cell.[1] In addition, the phosphorylation of a family of proteins located on the surface of the lipid droplet (perilipins) may be required before HSL can initiate lipolysis.[2] Perilipins create a barrier between HSL and cellular lipids and prevent lipolysis. Phosphorylation of perilipin allows HSL to gain access to intracellular triglycerides, possibly by modifying the surface of the lipid droplet.[3] The action of HSL on triglyceride yields 2 moles of unesterified fatty acids and 1 mole of monoglyceride. Hydrolysis of this remaining monoglyceride to one glycerol and one fatty acid moiety occurs readily through the action of monoglycerol lipase, which is not under direct hormonal control. Catecholamines (epinephrine and norepinephrine) and insulin are the major plasma hormones that regulate lipolysis in humans.

### 2.2.1   Adrenergic regulation of lipolysis

Catecholamines stimulate the lipolytic cascade by binding to β-adrenergic receptors ($\beta_1$, $\beta_2$, and $\beta_3$) on the cell surface, whereas catecholamine binding to $\alpha_2$-adrenergic receptors inhibits lipolytic activity. These receptors interact with membrane-bound guanosine triphosphate-binding regulatory proteins (G proteins), which modulate the activity of adenylate cyclase (see Figure 2.1). All β-adrenergic receptors are coupled with a stimulatory G protein known

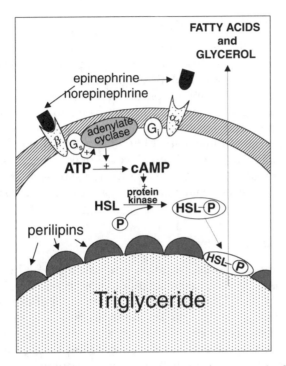

*Figure 2.1*   Schematic diagram representing the lipolytic cascade. β = beta-adrenergic receptor, $\alpha_2$ = alpha$_2$-adrenergic receptor, $G_s$ = stimulatory G protein, $G_i$ = inhibitory G protein, ATP = adenosine triphosphate, cAMP = cyclic adenosine monophosphate, HSL = hormone-sensitive lipase, and P = phosphate group.

as $G_s$, and $\alpha_2$-receptors are coupled with one or more of a group of inhibitory G proteins collectively known as $G_i$. Activation of adenylate cyclase by β-adrenergic stimulation catalyzes the conversion of adenosine triphosphate (ATP) to cyclic adenosine monophosphate (cAMP), thereby activating protein kinase, which then phosphorylates HSL and, presumably, perilipin.[2]

Catecholamines regulate lipolysis through stimulation of α- and β-adrenergic receptors; therefore, catecholamines can either increase or decrease lipolysis depending on catecholamine concentration and receptor binding affinity.[4] During exercise, the increase in circulating catecholamines stimulates lipolysis through β-adrenergic receptor activation.[5] The affinity for catecholamines differs among the three β-adrenergic receptors: $\beta_2 > \beta_1 > \beta_3$ for epinephrine, and $\beta_1 > \beta_2 > \beta_3$ for norepinephrine.[4,6] After prolonged exposure to catecholamines, β-adrenergic receptors become desensitized to catecholamine binding; however, each class of β-receptors differs in resistance to desensitization (i.e., $\beta_3 > \beta_2 > \beta_1$).[7] The receptor with the lowest affinity for catecholamines (i.e., $\beta_3$) remains active in response to prolonged catecholamine exposure and, therefore, may provide for more prolonged stimulation of lipolysis after the higher-affinity receptors have become desensitized.

## 2.2.2   Lipolytic regulation by insulin

Insulin is a potent inhibitor of lipolysis,[8] and a very small increase in plasma insulin concentration (i.e., 10–30 (U/mL) can suppress lipolytic rate to very low levels. Most of the antilipolytic action of insulin is due to stimulating the activity of one of the cellular phosphodiesterases[9] that degrade cAMP, thereby reducing the signaling cascade responsible for activating HSL. Insulin phosphorylates and subsequently activates phosphodiesterase through activation of phosphatidylinositol 3-kinase (PI3-K), which also plays a key role in mediating insulin-stimulated glucose uptake. Therefore, much of the effect of insulin on substrate metabolism (i.e., increase in carbohydrate metabolism and decrease in fat metabolism) appears to be through activation of PI3-K.

## 2.2.3   Regional lipolysis

Lipolytic activity differs among adipose tissue sites.[11,12] This variability in lipolytic rate is related to regional differences in adrenergic and insulin receptor density and function. Data from studies performed in isolated adipocytes indicate that lipolytic sensitivity to catecholamines is greater in fat cells obtained from intra-abdominal than subcutaneous adipose tissue.[13-15] Additionally, the antilipolytic effect of insulin is greater in fat cells obtained from subcutaneous than from intra-abdominal adipose tissue.[16] Although these data suggest that lipolytic activity is enhanced in adipocytes from intra-abdominal compared with subcutaneous fat, it is unlikely that intra-abdominal fat is an important contributor to fatty acid oxidation by skeletal muscle during exercise because this depot constitutes a very small portion of total body fat mass. Moreover, fatty acid release from the splanchnic region contributes only a very small portion to whole body fatty acid flux,[12] suggesting that most fatty acids released from this store may be cleared by the liver and never enter the systemic circulation. Therefore, most fatty acids delivered to skeletal muscle during exercise are derived from subcutaneous adipose tissue.

Lipolytic regulation is also heterogeneous among different subcutaneous adipose depots. Abdominal subcutaneous adipocytes are more sensitive to β-receptor agonists[17-20] and less sensitive to $\alpha_2$-receptor agonists[19,21] than adipocytes obtained from either femoral or gluteal adipose tissue. These differences in adipocyte β- and α-adrenergic sensitivity observed *in vitro* help explain region-specific differences in lipolytic sensitivity to catecholamines observed *in vivo*. For example, the increase in lipolytic rate that occurs during systemic epinephrine infusion *in vivo* is blunted in femoral compared with abdominal subcutaneous fat depots.[22] Moreover, during moderate-intensity endurance exercise, lipolysis of triglycerides is greater from upper-body than from lower-body fat subcutaneous adipose tissue.[23] Therefore, upper-body subcutaneous adipose tissue provides most of the fatty acids that are delivered to working muscles during exercise.

## 2.2.4   Adipose tissue blood flow

Adipose tissue blood flow helps regulate fatty acid release from adipose tissue by delivering lipolytic hormones and fatty acid carrier proteins (albumin) to adipose tissue and by exporting albumin-bound fatty acids from adipose tissue. Catecholamines stimulate β-adrenergic receptors in vascular smooth muscle within adipose and skeletal muscle, thereby reducing vascular tone and increasing blood flow. When plasma epinephrine concentrations are between 50 and 300 pg/mL, lipolysis and ATBF increase in parallel.[24] Therefore, during low- to moderate-intensity endurance exercise (25–65% maximal oxygen consumption, or $VO_2$max), when plasma epinephrine concentrations is <300 pg/mL, the coordinated increase of lipolysis and ATBF by catecholamines enhances the release of the newly liberated fatty acids from adipose tissue into the circulation, where they can be delivered to muscle for oxidation. Moderate-intensity exercise causes a twofold increase in adipose tissue blood flow[25,26] and more than a tenfold increase in muscle blood flow.

## 2.2.5   Other triglyceride sources

Other sources of triglycerides also contribute to fatty acid oxidation during endurance exercise. Intramuscular triglycerides (IMTGs) are lipid droplets stored within muscle cells, which can provide a considerable amount of fuel to muscle during exercise. IMTGs release fatty acids directly into the cytosol of working muscles.[26] Although the regulation of IMTG lipolysis during exercise is unclear, similarities have been found between IMTG and adipose tissue triglyceride lipolysis. For example, HSL has been isolated in skeletal muscle,[28] and stimulation of $β_2$-adrenergic receptors decrease IMTG content.[29] However, muscle HSL activity can also increase independently of adrenergic stimulation.[30] This increase in muscular HSL activity involves HSL phosphorylation, perhaps mediated by calcium release during muscle contraction.[29] Plasma triglycerides are another potential source of fuel for exercise.[31] Circulating triglycerides are hydrolyzed by lipoprotein lipase in the capillary endothelium of skeletal muscle and release fatty acids that can be taken up by muscle tissue. Although fatty acids derived from plasma triglycerides are not considered an important fuel during exercise, the contribution of circulating triglycerides to energy metabolism during exercise in humans has not been carefully studied.

# 2.3   Measurement of lipolysis

## 2.3.1   Whole-body lipolytic rate

The most reliable method for evaluating whole-body lipolytic rate during exercise involves measuring the dilution of infused labeled glycerol or fatty acid tracers in plasma. This approach provides an index of lipolysis by determining the rate of release of endogenous fatty acids or glycerol into the bloodstream. This methodology assumes that: (1) the breakdown of 1 mole of triglyceride releases 1 mole of glycerol and 3 moles of fatty acids into the bloodstream, and (2) all endogenous glycerol or fatty acids released into plasma will be detected by sampling peripheral blood during intravenous tracer infusion. However, these assumptions are not completely correct, and a clear understanding of the strengths and limitations of tracer methods is needed to properly interpret data from studies that have used isotope dilu-tion methods. Hydrolysis of adipose tissue triglycerides should release 1 mole of glycerol and 3 moles of fatty acids because partial hydrolysis of adipose tissue triglyceride is minimal.[32] Nearly all glycerol that is released during lipolysis enters the bloodstream because glycerol kinase, the enzyme needed to metabolize glycerol, is virtually absent in adipose tissue.[33] In contrast, fatty acids released during lipolysis can be re-esterified within adipose tissue without entering the bloodstream, which would cause an underestimation of lipolytic rate. Additionally, glycerol and fatty acids released into the portal vein from visceral adipose tissue, which are cleared by the liver, do not enter the systemic circulation and, therefore, are not detected by peripherally infused tracers. However, lipolysis of triglycerides present in visceral adipose tissue is likely to represent a very small percentage of whole-body lipolytic activity. The glycerol and fatty acid rates of appear-ance (Ra) in plasma, measured by isotope dilution methods, represent a summation of individual tissue events that release glycerol or fatty acids into the bloodstream, including lipolysis of different subcutaneous adipose tissue regions, intramuscular triglycerides, and plasma lipoproteins. The contribu-tion from each source may vary during different physiological conditions.

Whereas measurements of glycerol and fatty acid kinetics in blood pro-vide a reasonable representation of lipolytic rate, assessment of whole-body lipolysis by measuring concentrations of free fatty acid or glycerol in blood can be misleading because changes in plasma concentrations may not nec-essarily reflect changes in lipolytic rate. Plasma fatty acid or glycerol con-centration represents a balance between fatty acid or glycerol delivery into plasma and fatty acid or glycerol tissue uptake. The relationship between plasma fatty acid concentration and lipolysis can vary markedly depending on the physiological state.[34] For example, during endurance exercise, the change in plasma fatty acid concentrations may be minimal because both lipolytic rate (fatty acid release into plasma) and muscle oxidative require-ments for fatty acid (muscle uptake of plasma fatty acid) increase markedly. In contrast, epinephrine infusion at rest can cause marked increases in plasma fatty acid concentrations because the lipolysis is stimulated without a concomitant increase in muscle fatty acid uptake and oxidation.

### 2.3.2   Regional lipolytic rate

Local tissue lipolytic activity can be assessed *in vivo* by using standard arteriovenous principles, which involves evaluating the balance between the delivery (from an artery) and release (into a vein) of fatty acids or glycerol across an adipose tissue bed. This approach requires measurement of arterial and venous fatty acid or glycerol concentrations and ATBF. Subcutaneous ATBF can be determined by analyzing the clearance of $^{133}$Xe, an inert and lipophilic radioisotope that is injected locally into an adipose tissue bed.[35] Blood flow is quantified as the product of the fractional decline of $^{133}$Xe radioactivity at the site of injection and the partition coefficient for adipose tissue. Abdominal vein catheterization and microdialysis probe techniques permit the evaluation of regional fatty acids and/or glycerol released from adipose tissue.

Glycerol and fatty acids released into veins that drain blood from subcutaneous adipose tissue can be measured directly by sampling blood from an abdominal vein. This technique involves placing a small, 22-gauge catheter into an abdominal vein and positioning the tip so that it is superior to the inguinal ligament as judged by surface anatomy.[36] In this position, blood withdrawn from the catheter represents drainage from adipose tissue and overlying skin, without contribution from underlying muscle because the muscle is completely separated from the fat by a sheet of avascular fibrous tissue, which is the aponeurosis of the external oblique.[37] The microdialysis technique permits sampling of adipose tissue interstitial fluid. Microdialysis probes are placed percutaneously into subcutaneous abdominal adipose tissue. Each probe consists of dialysis tubing glued to the end of a double-steel cannula. Perfusion of a buffer solution (i.e., perfusate) through the inner cannula of the probe delivers perfusate into the space between the inner cannula and the outer dialysis membrane. The perfusate equilibrates with the fluid in the interstitial space surrounding the dialysis membrane and exits through the outer cannula for collection in small vials. Slow perfusion (0.03 mL/min) of Ringer's solution through the probe allows complete equilibration of interstitial glycerol with the perfusate,[38] so that the concentration of glycerol in collected perfusate is equal to the concentration of glycerol in the interstitium. Microdialysis data can be used to calculate regional glycerol Ra by converting interstitial glycerol concentrations (measured in microdialysis samples) to venous concentrations, based on Fick's law of diffusion for a thin membrane.[39]

## 2.4   Lipolytic response to exercise

### 2.4.1   Whole-body adipose tissue triglyceride lipolysis

During mild to moderate intensity exercise (i.e., 25–70% VO$_2$max), the rate of adipose tissue lipolysis increases two- to threefold above resting rates (see Figure 2.2).[40–42] In addition, the percentage of released fatty acids that are re-esterified decreases, and, therefore, a greater proportion of released fatty acids are delivered to skeletal muscle where they are oxidized.[41] Although whole-body lipolytic rate (measured as glycerol Ra) is maintained at a high rate as exercise intensity increases, fatty acid release into the circulation

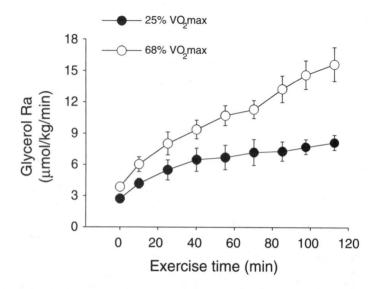

*Figure 2.2*    Whole-body lipolysis (glycerol Ra) during low-intensity (25% maximal oxygen uptake [VO₂max]) and moderate-intensity (68% VO₂max) exercise. (Adapted from Horowitz et al., *Am. J. Physiol.*, 276(5, part 1), E828, 1999.)

(measured as fatty acid Ra) and whole-body fat oxidation decline during high-intensity exercise.[43] The mechanism responsible for this phenomenon is not known but may be related to $\alpha_2$-adrenergic-mediated vasoconstriction at high plasma catecholamine concentrations, which decreases ATBF and may suppress fatty acid release into the systemic circulation.[44] This reduction in fatty acid availability may help explain why fat oxidation is suppressed during high-intensity exercise. In fact, increasing plasma fatty acid concentration during high-intensity exercise by infusing a lipid emulsion and heparin has been found to increase total fat oxidation by about 30%.[45-47] However, fat oxidation was not completely restored to the rate observed during moderate-intensity exercise.[43,45] Therefore, fat oxidation during high-intensity exercise is limited by both a decreased plasma fatty acid availability and alterations in fatty acid metabolism within muscle itself.[48]

### 2.4.2   Regional adipose tissue triglyceride lipolysis

During steady-state endurance exercise, the lipolytic rate increases progressively in abdominal but not femoral/gluteal subcutaneous adipose tissue;[5,23] therefore, it is likely that most of the plasma fatty acids available to working muscle are derived from upper-body rather than lower-body subcutaneous fat. This is consistent with studies demonstrating regional differences in lipolytic sensitivity to catecholamines *in vivo*[18] and *in vitro*.[20] It is likely that differences in local adipose tissue $\alpha_2$- and $\beta$-adrenergic receptor affinity, density, and function[20] are responsible for regional heterogeneity in an exercise-induced lipolytic rate.

### 2.4.3   Carbohydrate ingestion

Carbohydrate ingestion elicits an antilipolytic effect on adipose tissue by increasing plasma insulin concentration. Ingestion of only a small carbohydrate load during the hour before exercise reduces lipolysis sufficiently to limit fatty acid oxidation during a subsequent exercise bout.[49] Consequently, muscle glycogen oxidation increases during the early portion of exercise to compensate for the reduction in energy derived from fat. Adipose tissue lipolysis is even sensitive to the small insulin response caused by ingestion of low-glycemic carbohydrates, such as fructose (see Figure 2.3).[49] Although the duration of the influence of insulin on lipolysis is not known, the normal increase in fat oxidation during exercise can be blunted up to 6 hours after a meal;[51] therefore, during normal daily living conditions, lipolytic rate during exercise is often influenced by the insulin response to the meal ingested in the hours before an exercise bout.

Carbohydrate ingestion during endurance exercise can delay fatigue by providing exogenous glucose as a fuel late in exercise when endogenous glycogen stores are very low;[52] however, carbohydrate ingestion also decreases endogenous substrate availability by suppressing lipolytic rate. Nonetheless, lipolytic rate after carbohydrate ingestion during exercise does not limit fat oxidation because plasma fatty acid availability exceeds plasma fatty acid oxidation.[40]

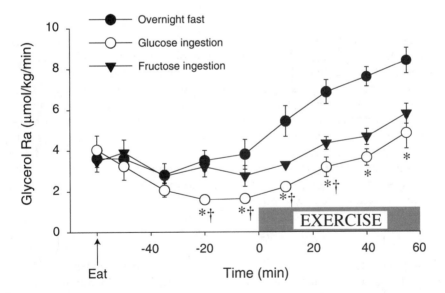

*Figure 2.3*    Whole-body lipolytic response (glycerol Ra) at rest and during exercise after ingestion of ~60 g of carbohydrate from either glucose or fructose; * indicates significantly different than overnight fast ($p < 0.05$), and † indicates significantly different than fructose ingestion ($p < 0.05$). (Adapted from Horowitz et al., *Am. J. Physiol.*, 273(36), E768, 1997.)

## 2.4.4   Obesity

Although basal lipolytic rate is greater in persons with upper-body (abdominal) obesity compared with lower-body obese and lean persons,[12] lipolytic sensitivity to catecholamines is blunted in persons with abdominal obesity.[11,53] This blunted lipolytic sensitivity has been attributed to a low density of $\beta_2$-adrenergic receptors in adipocytes from subcutaneous abdominal adipose tissue.[54] Moreover, a blunted lipolytic response to catecholamines in subcutaneous fat of the abdomen but not the femoral region has been demonstrated *in vivo*.[22] Because $\beta$-adrenergic stimulation is largely responsible for the exercise-induced increase in lipolysis,[5] the suppressed lipolytic sensitivity may be responsible for the blunted increase in fatty acid mobilization during exercise in persons with abdominal obesity. However, only the incremental increase in lipolysis is blunted; the absolute rate of fatty acid mobilization is similar in lean and obese subjects during exercise.[55,56]

Despite similar rates of fatty acid release into plasma, the source of fatty acids used during exercise differs in lean and obese subjects.[56] The authors have recently found that although uptake and oxidation of circulating fatty acids were similar in lean and abdominally obese women during exercise, fat oxidation was 25% greater in obese subjects.[56] Therefore, persons with abdominal obesity must oxidize a greater proportion of an alternative source of fatty acids, presumably those derived from IMTGs.

## 2.4.5   Aging

Lipolysis and fatty acid release into plasma is greater in older (>70 years) compared with younger (<35 years) adults exercising at the same absolute intensity.[57] Despite this enhanced fatty acid availability, fat oxidation is lower in older than in younger subjects,[57] presumably due to alterations in skeletal muscle fatty acid metabolism. Consistent with this notion, mitochondrial oxidative capacity has been found to be reduced in muscle homogenates from older compared with younger subjects.[58] Endurance exercise training in elderly subjects increases muscle oxidative capacity and fat oxidation without altering fatty acid release into the circulation;[57] therefore, poor aerobic fitness, which impairs muscle fatty acid oxidative capacity, contributes to the low rate of fat oxidation observed with advancing age.

## 2.5   Endurance exercise training

Endurance training increases the use of fat as a fuel during exercise;[59] however, the increase in fat oxidation is not due to increased mobilization of adipose tissue triglycerides. Lipolytic rates are similar in endurance-trained athletes and untrained volunteers during exercise performed at the same absolute intensity.[42] Additionally, data from longitudinal studies indicate that several weeks of endurance training does not increase[23] (and may even decrease[60,61]) plasma fatty acid mobilization during exercise, which is likely due to a suppressed catecholamine response to exercise after training. These data suggest that the increase in fatty acid oxidation observed after training is derived from a source other than circulating fatty acids. The results from several studies suggest that the increase in fat oxidation after endurance training is due to an increase in IMTG oxidation;[23,60–62] however, the precise source of the additional oxidized fatty acids is controversial because of the technical difficulties in directly assessing the oxidation of IMTGs.

Although data from several studies have found that the maximal lipolytic response to epinephrine (concentrations between $10^{-6}$ and $10^{-4}$ mol/L) is greater in isolated adipocytes obtained from endurance-trained than in those from untrained subjects.[63–66] At physiologic epinephrine concentrations (between $10^{-10}$ and $10^{-8}$ mol/L), lipolytic activity is the same or slightly lower in adipocytes from endurance-trained subjects compared with those from untrained subjects.[64,65] Similarly, Stallknecht et al.[67] found that the lipolytic response of abdominal subcutaneous adipose tissue to epinephrine infusion *in vivo* was the same in trained and untrained subjects. Moreover, in a longitudinal study, the authors have found that whole-body lipolytic sensitivity to a physiologic range of epinephrine concentrations was not affected by endurance training (see Figure 2.4).[24] Therefore, although the maximal lipolytic response to catecholamines *in vitro* is enhanced by endurance training, lipolytic sensitivity to catecholamines, across a physiological range of plasma epinephrine concentrations *in vivo*, remains unchanged.

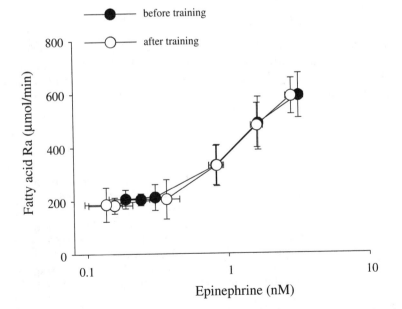

*Figure 2.4*    The effect of endurance exercise training on fatty acid rate of appearance (fatty acid Ra) in plasma in response to a physiological range of plasma epinephrine concentrations. (Adapted from Horowitz et al., *Am. J. Physiol.*, 277(40), E325, 1999.)

During exercise performed at the same relative intensity (i.e., same %VO$_2$max), the whole-body lipolytic rate (glycerol Ra) is greater in endurance-trained than in untrained persons.[68,69] The mechanism responsible for the higher rate of lipolysis in trained subjects is not clear but may be related to both the greater absolute intensity of exercise being performed and enhanced contraction-mediated IMTG lipolysis. In addition, endurance-trained athletes have a greater adipose tissue blood flow in response to epinephrine infusion compared with sedentary control subjects.[67] Thus, catecholamine delivery to adipose tissue may be greater during exercise.

## 2.6   Summary and conclusions

Adipose tissue triglycerides are an important source of fuel during exercise. The increase in lipolytic rate and availability of fatty acids that occurs during exercise requires the integration of neural, hormonal, and circulatory events, which facilitate delivery of fatty acids from adipose tissue to skeletal muscle mitochondria for oxidation. During endurance exercise, lipolysis of adipose tissue triglycerides is heterogeneous and is greater in upper-body than in lower-body subcutaneous fat depots. Age, body fat content, nutritional state, and aerobic fitness can affect the mobilization and/or oxidation of adipose tissue triglycerides and, therefore, the mix of fuels that are used to provide energy for working muscles during exercise.

## Acknowledgments

This research was supported by National Institutes of Health grants DK-37948, DK-56341 (Clinical Nutrition Research Unit), RR-0036 (General Clinical Research Center), RR-00954, (Mass Spectrometry Resource), AG-13629 (Claude Pepper Older American Independence Center), and AG-00078 (Institutional National Research Service Award).

## References

1.  Egan, J.J., Greenberg, A.S., Chang, M.K. et al., Mechanism of hormone-stimulated lipolysis in adipocytes: translocation of hormone-sensitive lipase to the lipid storage droplet, *Proc. Natl. Acad. Sci.*, 89(18), 8537, 1992.
2.  Londos, C., Brasaemle, D.L., Gruia-Gray, J. et al., Perilipin: unique proteins associated with intracellular muetral lipid droplets in adipocytes and steroidogenic cells, *Biochem. Soc. Trans.*, 23(3), 611, 1995.
3.  Souza, S.C., Moitoso de Vargas, L., Yamamoto, M.T. et al., Overexpression of perilipin A and B blocks the ability of tumor necrosis factor to increase lipolysis in 3T3-L1 adipocytes, *J. Biol. Chem.*, 273(38), 24665, 1998.
4.  Galitzky, J., Reverte, M., Portillo, M. et al., Coexistence of $\beta_1$-, $\beta_2$-, and $\beta_3$-adrenoceptors in dog fat cells and their differential activation by catecholamines, *Am. J. Physiol.*, 264(3, part 1), E402, 1993.

5. Arner, P., Kriegholm, E., Engfeldt, P. et al., Adrenergic regulation of lipolysis in situ at rest and during exercise, *J. Clin. Invest.*, 85, 893, 1990.

6. Lafontan, M., Bousquet-Melou, A., Galitzky, J. et al., Adrenergic receptors and fat cells: differential recruitment by physiological amines and homologous regulation, *Obesity Res.*, 3(suppl. 4), 507S, 1995.

7. Granneman, J.G., Why do adipocytes make the $\beta_3$ adrenergic receptor? *Cell Sig.*, 7(1), 9, 1995.

8. Campbell, P.J., Carlson, M.G., Hill, J.O. et al., Regulation of free fatty acid metabolism by insulin in humans: role of lipolysis and reesterification, *Am. J. Physiol.*, 26, E1063, 1992.

9. Eriksson, H., Ridderstrale, M., Degerman, E. et al., Evidence for the key role of the adipocyte cGMP-inhibited cAMP phosphodiesterase in the antilipolytic action of insulin, *Biochim. Biophys. Acta*, 1266(1), 101, 1995.

10. Rahn, T., Ridderstrale, M., Tornqvist, H. et al., Essential role of phosphatidylinositol 3-kinase in insulin-induced activation and phosphorylation of the cGMP-inhibited cAMP phosphodiesterase in rat adipocytes. Studies using the selective inhibitor wortmannin, *FEBS Lett.*, 350(2–3), 314, 1994.

11. Jensen, M.D., Haymond, M.W., Rizza, R.A. et al., Influence of body fat distribution on free fatty acid metabolism in obesity, *J. Clin. Invest.*, 83, 1168, 1989.

12. Martin, M.L. and Jensen, M.D., Effects of body fat distribution on regional lipolysis in obesity, *J. Clin. Invest.*, 88, 609, 1991.

13. Hellmer, J., Marcus, C., Sonnenfeld, T. et al., Mechanisms for differences in lipolysis between human subcutaneous and omental fat cells, *J. Clin. Endocrinol. Metab.*, 75(1), 15, 1992.

14. Mauriege, P., Galitzky, J., Berlan, M. et al., Heterogeneous distribution of $\beta$- and $\alpha_2$-adrenoceptor binding sites in human fat cells from various fat deposits: functional consequences, *Eur J. Clin. Invest.*, 17(2), 156, 1987.

15. Rebuffe-Scrive, M., Lonnroth, P., Marin, P. et al., Regional adipose tissue metabolism in men and postmenopausal women, *Int. J. Obesity*, 11(4), 347, 1987.

16. Richelsen, B., Pedersen, S.B., Moller-Pedersen, T. et al., Regional differences in triglyceride breakdown in human adipose tissue: effects of catecholamines, insulin, and prostaglandin E2, *Metabolism*, 40(9), 990, 1991.

17. Berman, D., Nicklas, B., Rogus, E. et al., Regional differences in adrenceptor binding and fat cell lipolysis in obese, postmenopausal women, *Metabolism*, 47(4), 467, 1998.

18. Guo, Z., Johnson, C.M., and Jensen, M.D., Regional lipolytic responses to isoproterenol in women, *Am. J. Physiol.*, 273(36), E108, 1997.

19. Rosenbaum, M., Presta, E., Hirsch, J. et al., Regional differences in adrenoreceptor status of adipose tissue in adults and prepubertal children, *J. Clin. Endocrinol. Metab.*, 73(2), 341, 1991.

20. Wahrenberg, H., Lonnqvist, F., and Arner, P., Mechanisms underlying regional differences in lipolysis in human adipose tissue, *J. Clin. Invest.*, 84, 458, 1989.

21. Lafontan, M., Dang-Tran, L., and Berlan, M., Alpha-adrenergic antilipolytic effect of adrenaline in human fat cells of the thigh: comparison with adrenaline responsiveness of different fat deposits, *Eur. J. Clin. Invest.*, 9(4), 261, 1979.

22. Horowitz, J.F. and Klein, S., Whole body and abdominal lipolytic sensitivity to epinephrine is suppressed in upper body obese women, *Am. J. Physiol.*, 278, E1144, 2000.

23. Horowitz, J.F., Leone, T.C., Feng, W. et al., Effect of endurance training on lipid metabolism in women: a potential role for PPARa in the metabolic response to training, *Am. J. Physiol.*, 279, E348, 2000.

24. Horowitz, J.F., Braudy, R.J., Martin, W.H. et al., Endurance exercise training does not alter lipolytic or adipose tissue blood flow sensitivity to epinephrine, *Am. J. Physiol.*, 277(40), E325, 1999.

25. Bulow, J. and Madsen, J., Adipose tissue blood flow during prolonged, heavy exercise, *Pflüg. Arch.*, 363, 231, 1976.

26. Bulow, J. and Madsen, J., Influence of blood flow on fatty acid mobilization from lipolytically active tissue, *Pflüg. Arch.*, 390, 169–174, 1981.

27. Carlson, L.A., Eklund, L.G., and Froberg, S.O., Concentration of triglycerides, phospholipids, and glycogen in skeletal muscle and of free fatty acids and β-hydroxybutyric acid in blood in man in response to exercise, *Eur. J. Clin. Invest.*, 1, 248, 1971.

28. Langfort, J., Ploug, T., Ihlemann, J. et al., Expression of hormone-sensitive lipase and its regulation by adrenaline in skeletal muscle, *Biochem. J.*, 340, 459, 1999.

29. Cleroux, J., Van Ngnyen, P., Taylor, A.W. et al., Effects of $\beta_1$- vs. $\beta_1+\beta_2$-blockade on exercise endurance and muscle metabolism in humans, *J. Appl. Physiol.*, 66, 548, 1989.

30. Langfort, J., Ploug, T., Ihlemann, J. et al., Stimulation of hormone-sensitive lipase activity by contractions in rat skeletal muscle, *Biochem. J.*, 351, 1, 207, 2000.

31. Olsson, A.G., Eklund, B., Kaijser, L. et al., Extraction of exogenous plasma triglycerides by the working human forearm muscle in the fasting state, *Scand. J. Clin. Invest.*, 35, 231, 1975.

32. Arner, P. and Ostman, J., Mono- and diacylglycerols in human adipose tissue, *Biochim. Biophys. Acta*, 369, 209, 1974.

33. Lin, E.C.C., Glycerol utilization and its regulation in mammals, *Annual Review of Biochemistry*, 46, 765, 1977.

34. Klein, S., Coyle, E.F., and Wolfe, R.R., Effect of exercise on lipolytic sensitivity in endurance-trained athletes, *J. Appl. Physiol.*, 78(6), 2201, 1995.

35. Larsen, O.A., Lassen, N.A., and Quaade, F., Blood flow through human adipose tissue determined with radioactive xenon, *Acta Physiol. Scand.*, 66, 337, 1966.

36. Frayn, K.N., Coppack, S.W., and Humphreys, S.M., Subcutaneous adipose tissue metabolism studied by local catheterization, *Int. J. Obesity*, 17(suppl. 3), S18, 1993.

37. Frayn, K.N., Coppack, S.W., Humphreys, S.M. et al., Metabolic characteristics of human adipose tissue in vivo, *Clin. Sci. (Colch.)*, 76(5), 509, 1989.

38. Rosdahl, H., Hamrin, K., Ungerstedt, U. et al., Metabolite levels in human skeletal muscle and adipose tissue studied with microdialysis at low perfusion flow, *Am. J. Physiol.*, 274(37), E936, 1998.

39. Intaglietta, M. and Johnson, P.C., Principles of capillary exchange, in *Principles of Capillary Exchange*, P.C. Johnson, Ed., John Wiley & Sons, New York, 1978, p. 141.

40. Horowitz, J.F., Mora-Rodriguez, R., Byerley, L.O. et al., Substrate metabolism when subjects are fed carbohydrates during exercise, *Am. J. Physiol.*, 276(5, part 1), E828, 1999.

41. Wolfe, R.R., Klein, S., Carraro, F. et al., Role of triglyceride-fatty acid cycle in controlling fat metabolism in humans during and after exercise, *Am. J. Physiol.*, 258(21), E382, 1990.

42. Klein, S., Coyle, E.F., and Wolfe, R.R., Fat metabolism during low-intensity exercise in endurance trained and untrained men, *Am. J. Physiol. (Endocrinol. Metab.)*, 267(30), E934, 1994.

43. Romijn, J.A., Coyle, E.F., Sidossis, L. et al., Regulation of endogenous fat and carbohydrate metabolism in relation to exercise intensity, *Am. J. Physiol.*, 265(28), E380, 1993.

44. Hodgetts, V., Coppack, S.W., Frayn, K.N. et al., Factors controlling fat mobilization from human subcutaneous adipose tissue during exercise, *J. Appl. Physiol.*, 71(2), 445, 1991.

45. Romijn, J.A., Coyle, E.F., Zhang, X.-J. et al., Fat oxidation is impaired somewhat during high-intensity exercise by limited plasma FFA mobilization, *J. Appl. Physiol.*, 79(6), 1939, 1995.

46. Vukovich, M.D., Costill, D.L., Hickey, M.S. et al., Effect of fat emulsion infusion and fat feeding on muscle glycogen utilization during cycle exercise, *J. Appl. Physiol.*, 75(4), 1513, 1993.

47. Dyck, D.J., Putman, C.T., Heigenhauser, J.F. et al., Regulation of fat-carbohydrate interaction in skeletal muscle during intense aerobic cycling, *Am. J. Physiol.*, 265(28), E852, 1993.

48. Sidossis, L.S., Gastaldelli, A., Klein, S. et al., Regulation of plasma fatty acid oxidation during low- and high-intensity exercise, *Am. J. Physiol.*, 272(35), E1065, 1997.

49. Horowitz, J.F., Mora-Rodriguez, R., Byerley, L.O. et al., Lipolytic suppression following carbohydrate ingestion limits fat oxidation during exercise, *Am. J. Physiol.*, 273(36), E768, 1997.

50. Gollnick, P.D., Pernow, B., Essen, B. et al., Availability of glycogen and plasma FFA for substrate utilization in leg muscle of man, *Clin. Physiol.*, 1, 27, 1981.

51. Montain, S.J., Hopper, M.K., Coggan, A.R. et al., Exercise metabolism at different time intervals after a meal, *J. Appl. Physiol.*, 70(2), 882, 1991.

52. Coyle, E.F., Coggan, A.R., Hemmert, M.K. et al., Muscle glycogen utilization during prolonged strenuous exercise when fed carbohydrates, *J. Appl. Physiol.*, 61, 165, 1986.

53. Connacher, A.A., Bennet, W.M., Jung, R.T. et al., Effect of adrenaline infusion on fatty acid and glucose turnover in lean and obese human subjects in the post-absorptive and fed states, *Clin. Sci.*, 81, 635, 1991.

54. Reynisdottir, S., Wahrenberg, H., Calstrom, K. et al., Catecholamine resistance in fat cells of women with upper-body obesity due to decreased expression of $\beta_2$-adrenoceptors, *Diabetologia*, 37, 428, 1994.

55. Kanaley, J.A., Cryer, P.E., and Jensen, M.D., Fatty acid kinetic responses to exercise. Effects of obesity, body fat distribution, and energy-restricted diet, *J. Clin. Invest.*, 92(1), 255, 1993.

56. Horowitz, J.F. and Klein, S., Oxidation of nonplasma fatty acids during exercise is increased in women with abdominal obesity, *J. Appl. Physiol.*, 89, 2276, 2000.

57. Sial, S., Coggan, A., Carroll, R. et al., Fat and carbohydrate metabolism during exercise in elderly and young subjects, *Am. J. Physiol.*, 271(34), E983, 1996.

58. Morio, B., Hocquette, J.F., Montaurier, C. et al., Muscle fatty acid oxidative capacity is a determinant of whole-body fat oxidation in elderly people, *Am. J. Physiol. (Endocrinol. Metab.)*, 280(1), E143, 2001.

59. Holloszy, J.O. and Coyle, E.F., Adaptations of skeletal muscle to endurance exercise and their metabolic consequences, *J. Appl. Physiol.*, 56, 831, 1984.

60. Martin, W.H.I., Dalsky, G.P., Hurley, B.F. et al., Effect of endurance training on plasma free fatty acid turnover and oxidation during exercise, *Am. J. Physiol. (Endocrinol. Metab.)*, 265(28), E708, 1996.

61. Phillips, S.M., Green, H.J., Tarnopolsky, M.A. et al., Effects of training duration on substrate turnover and oxidation during exercise, *J. Appl. Physiol.*, 81(5), 2182, 1996.

62. Hurley, B.F., Nemeth, P.M., Martin, W.H. et al., Muscle triglyceride utilization during exercise: effect of training, *J. Appl. Physiol.*, 60(2), 562, 1986.

63. Despres, J.P., Bouchard, C., Savard, R. et al., The effect of a 20-week endurance training program on adipose-tissue morphology and lipolysis in men and women, *Metabolism*, 33(3), 235, 1984.

64. Crampes, F., Beauville, M., Riviere, D. et al., Effect of physical training in humans on the response of isolated fat cells to epinephrine, *J. Appl. Physiol.*, 61(1), 25, 1986.

65. Crampes, F., Riviere, D., Beauville, M. et al., Lipolytic response of adipocytes to epinephrine in sedentary and exercise-trained subjects: sex-related differences, *Eur. J. Appl. Physiol.*, 59, 249, 1989.

66. Riviere, D., Crampes, F., Beauville, M. et al., Lipolytic response of fat cells to catecholamines in sedentary and exercise-trained women, *J. Appl. Physiol.*, 66(1), 330, 1989.

67. Stallknecht, B., Simonsen, L., Bulow, J. et al., Effect of training on epinephrine-stimulated lipolysis determined by microdialysis in human adipose tissue, *Am. J. of Physiol. (Endocrinol. Metab.)*, 269(32), E1059, 1995.

68. Klein, S., Weber, J.M., Coyle, E.F. et al., Effect of endurance training on glycerol kinetics during strenuous exercise in humans, *Metabolism*, 43(3), 357, 1996.

69. Coggan, A.R., Raguso, C.A., Gastaldelli, A. et al., Fat metabolism during high-intensity exercise in endurance-trained and untrained men, *Metabolism*, 49(1), 122, 2000.

*chapter three*

# Endurance exercise effects on adipose tissue lipoprotein lipase

**Richard L. Seip**

## Contents

## 3.1   Introduction

The physiologically active form of the enzyme lipoprotein lipase (LPL, EC
3.1.1.34) is found anchored to the endothelial cells of the capillary lumen,[1]
in and near the tissues of its origin. Here it catalyzes the hydrolysis of plasma
lipoprotein triglycerides, yielding free fatty acids for uptake by the local
tissues. Tissue-specific regulation of LPL activity (LPLA) directs lipoprotein-
triglyceride-derived free fatty acids to appropriate tissues. Because adipose
tissue LPLA (expressed per unit tissue mass) exceeds that of skeletal muscle
by three- to tenfold in rat[2] or mouse[3] and by one- to fourfold in man,[4] normal
resting conditions in the healthy, fed, sedentary mammals favor fatty acid
distribution to adipose tissue for storage.

Adipose tissue lipoprotein lipase is interesting for several reasons. First,
it is a suspected regulator of obesity. Second, LPLA within the circulation
decreases plasma triglycerides,[5] alters the size and lipid composition of
plasma-triglyceride-rich lipoproteins,[6] and elevates the concentration of
plasma high-density lipoprotein cholesterol.[7] All of these processes lower
cardiovascular disease risk.[8] Finally, tissue LPLA may help control the size
of regional adipose depots.[9] The role of exercise in all of these has been
investigated.

Exercise is an act of the muscles requiring a great increase in metabolic
rate. In response, muscle expresses proteins that participate in fuel procure-
ment, including glucose transport protein 4 (GLUT-4)[10] and LPL.[11–13] In contrast, adipose tissue (AT) metabolism does not increase during exercise,[14,15]
and the exercise increase in AT blood flow is far less than skeletal muscle.[15,16]
In adipose tissue, blood flow increases more with eating than exercise,[14] and
a change in food intake status (eating, fasting, and starvation) stimulates a

greater change in AT LPL compared to exercise. In fact, *in vivo*, many factors besides the exercise bout type and length — such as eating, fitness level, body composition (obesity and adipocyte size), regional site, gender, presence/absence of insulin resistance, and LPL genotype — have been investigated in relation to adipose LPL. This chapter considers the effects of exercise on adipose tissue lipoprotein lipase activity in the context of these factors and discusses mechanisms of LPL regulation.

## 3.2 Measurement of lipoprotein lipase

Tissue LPLA has been studied as physiologically separate fractions: heparin-releasable (HR) and that which is non-heparin-releasable. The non-heparin-releasable fraction is sometimes called "tissue-bound," "tissue-extractable" (EXT),[17] or "residual."[18] The heparin-releasable lipoprotein lipase activity (HR-LPLA) pool is thought to represent the mature, physiologically active LPL attached to the capillary endothelial cells, while the EXT fraction is thought to represent the sum of the activities of pools of precursor at various stages of maturation. The most popular assay methods use radiolabeled triglyceride emulsions as substrates, as described in primary references[4,19] and reviews.[20,21] In this method, the HR-LPL is obtained by allowing small pieces of adipose tissue to incubate, usually for 30 min at 28 to 37°C in a solution containing heparin, which elutes a fraction of the total LPL from the tissue.[20] The tissue-extractable LPL (EXT-LPL) pool is obtained after heparin incubation by homogenizing the washed tissue in detergent, then assaying the infranatant after centrifugation of the homogenate. Total LPLA, designated LPLTA in this chapter, and total LPL mass are derived from whole tissue pieces homogenized without incubation. Because of convenience and the belief that it represents the most physiologically relevant LPL fraction, HR-LPLA is most commonly measured. Under standard assay conditions, subcutaneous AT HR-LPLA in humans represents 30 to 60% of LPLTA,[17,22] but HR-LPL mass constitutes only 10 to 30% of AT total LPL immunoreactive content.[22,23]

## 3.3 Cross-sectional studies: comparing populations with different exercise habits

### 3.3.1 Pioneering studies

Early studies of LPL in humans were of subcutaneous adipose tissue from endurance-trained athletes. In 1978, Nikkila and colleagues[24] reported both higher adipose and skeletal muscle tissue HR-LPLA in competitive runners compared with controls. In endurance athletes but not sprinters, HR-LPLA of subcutaneous gluteal adipose tissue was 2.7-fold higher in men and 44% higher in women.[24] Marniemi et al.[25] found 70% higher abdominal AT LPLA in trained athletes vs. controls, though this was barely significant due to wide inter-individual variation. Peltonen et al.[26]

reported a modest correlation ($r = 0.38$) between abdominal AT LPLA and physical activity patterns in young men. In suprailiac tissue of near-elite marathoners who fasted for 12 hr, Savard et al.[27] found that the adipocyte diameter was 14% smaller in runners compared with sedentary but lean controls. In the runners, AT HR-LPLA was 60% higher when expressed per gram of tissue and 80 to 90% higher when expressed per cell diameter. These findings imply that endurance training in humans might increase AT LPLA. Additionally, in runners, Nikkila et al.[24] found that elevated blood high-density lipoprotein cholesterol (HDL-C) (a prominent cardio-vascular disease risk factor) was strongly predicted by elevated AT lipo-protein activity ($r = 0.94$). This finding especially sparked interest among exercise scientists.

### 3.3.2   Recent studies

Results of recent cross-sectional studies differ. In older men (mean age, 61 years), Berman et al.[28] found AT HR-LPLA to be 70 to 76% lower in runners compared with obese men, and 11 to 38% lower in runners compared with lean men. Adipocytes (mean cell triglyceride or TG mass, 0.22 to 0.27 µg) in runners were roughly half the size of the obese men's adipocytes and 20 to 30% smaller than those of the lean men. Tissue samples were obtained 24 to 36 hr post-exercise. In contrast to an earlier study,[24] abdominal AT HR-LPLA was negatively related ($r = -0.32$) and gluteal AT HR-LPLA was unrelated to plasma HDL-C. Controlling for percent body fat eliminated the significance.

In women, the data are also conflicting. Mauriege et al.[29] reported 36% lower subcutaneous femoral and 60% lower abdominal AT HR-LPLA (expressed per cell surface area) in endurance-trained compared with seden-tary women. The women were matched for body mass index (BMI) but differed in body fat (20% for the trained vs. 27% for the control women) and cardiorespiratory capacity (53 vs. 32 mL $O_2$ kg$^{-1}$ min$^{-1}$). Compared to controls, the fat-cell size of the trained women was 45% smaller at the abdominal site and 21% smaller at the femoral site. The runners were inactive for the pre-vious 60 hr. Because the rates of lipolysis in the adipocytes harvested from the runners were higher, Mauriege et al.[29] concluded that endurance-trained women showed a preferential lipid mobilization from the abdominal depot.

## 3.4   Acute exercise effect

### 3.4.1   Acute endurance exercise: bout intensity and duration

In human adipose tissue, subcutaneous AT HR-LPL can rise following a single bout of exercise, but this depends on the duration (and energy require-ment) of the bout, the exercise capacity of the subject, and perhaps adipocyte size. In rats, AT.LPL clearly decreases. In rats, usually internal adipose tissues have been sampled; it is not entirely clear if the difference between humans and rats is a species difference or a depot effect.

### 3.4.1.1  Rats

In 1963, Nikkila et al.[30] reported a 48% decrease in epididymal AT HR-LPLA, and increases of 66% in the myocardium and 28% in skeletal muscle following 60 minutes of treadmill running. The decrease in AT LPLA extends to 24 hr post-exercise. Barakat et al.[31] found a decrease (29% immediate and 47% at 24 hr post-exercise) in epididymal AT LPLTA in untrained male Hultsman rats that were treadmill-exercised to exhaustion (115 ± 10 min). The decrease is absent in epididymal fat of untrained diabetic male Wistar rats. Normal rats decreased LPLA by 23% immediately post-exercise and by 75% at 24 hr, while LPLA of diabetic rats fell 51% immediately post-exercise and 17% at 24 hr.[32]

Lambert et al.[33] reported marked increases in epididymal AT HR-LPLA following acute, high-intensity exercise to exhaustion, confirming an earlier similar report.[34] Sedentary, trained, and 1- and 2-week detrained rats were exercised on the treadmill until exhaustion (means, 21.5 min for sedentary and 27.8 min for trained). Acute exhaustive exercise failed to alter AT HR-LPLA in sedentary animals; however, it rose by 240% in trained animals and by 150% in the 1- and 2-week detrained animals. Differences from previous studies include the measurement of HR-LPLA vs. LPLTA and the use of exhaustive, high-intensity exercise. A possible explanation is that high-intensity exercise releases catecholamines that could alter the AT LPL response. Epinephrine infusion *in vivo* increases HR-LPLA measured *in vitro*.[35]

Few studies have examined the mechanism underlying the decrease in AT LPLA in rats. In sedentary male Wistar rats, Paulin et al.[36] found 40% and 58% decreases in epididymal white AT LPLTA and interscapular brown AT LPLTA, respectively, and decreases of 53% and 30%, respectively, in skeletal muscle and cardiac muscle. Nadolol (25 mg kg$^{-1}$ day$^{-1}$), a nonselective beta-blocker, did not affect the tissue responses. The authors concluded that the immediate response to exercise is independent of the β-adrenergic pathway. Another study showed that the rise in serum free fatty acids during exercise does not affect AT LPL.[37] LaDu et al.[38] investigated the LPL mRNA responses to exercise in the rat. They reported a significant 43% decrease in epididymal AT LPLTA in rats immediately following 2 hr of swimming. LPL mRNA fell 42%, suggesting transcriptional regulation. In the following 24 hr, animals ate freely and LPLTA recovered to within 14% of pre-exercise, but LPL mRNA remained 23% lower than pre-exercise,[38] suggesting post-translational regulation.

### 3.4.1.2  Humans

Long endurance bouts performed by lean subjects with high fitness levels acutely raise subcutaneous abdominal AT HR-LPLA by 20 to 45% (see Table 3.1).[39–42] The rise in AT LPL is a fraction of that seen in exercising skeletal muscle, which can increase by twofold in these subjects.[42] Thus, rats and fit humans differ in AT LPL response to acute exercise. In rats, endurance exercise decreases AT LPLA — a change designed to spare lipoprotein-derived

**Table 3.1**　Effect of Acute Exercise on Adipose Tissue Lipoprotein Lipase Activity in Trained Subjects

| Study | Subjects | Adipose Tissue Sample Site | Conditions | Exercise Bout | AT LPL Findings | Authors' Interpretation | Comments |
|---|---|---|---|---|---|---|---|
| Taskinen et al.[42] | n = 10 males; trained, lean; ages 17–42 | Subcutaneous gluteal | Morning, fasted | 20-km run lasting 85–105 min | 20% increase in HR-LPLA ($p < 0.05$) | — | Skeletal muscle HR-LPLA increased 110% |
| Lithell et al.[39] | n = 1 female, 6 males; healthy; ages 22–28 | Subcutaneous abdominal | Exercise in p.m. after 6 hr of normal eating (breakfast and lunch) | 1 hr at 63–68% of HR maximum (heart rate >190 beats/min at end of bout) | 44% increase in HR-LPLA ($p < 0.05$) | Feeding raised insulin; the fall in insulin with exercise was too short to effect up-regulation of HR-LPL in adipose tissue; thus, adipose tissue LPL rose due to feeding | Skeletal muscle HR-LPLA fell 15% |
| Savard et al.[40] | n = 27 healthy moderately active men (age 21.1±3.2, %BF 11.8 ± 5.1%, VO$_2$ max 50.9±5.8). | Subcutaneous suprailiac | Exercise 90 min after a light (560 kcal), mostly carbohydrate meal | Maximum sustainable cycle work for 90 min, resulting in 88% of maximum heart rate by the end of the bout | 28% increase in HR-LPLA per tissue mass; 37% increase per cell | Meal contributed only marginally to the rise; physiologic implication of AT LPL rise: raise blood FFA concentration for skeletal muscle uptake | No skeletal muscle data; adipocyte size was small (0.332 µg) |

fatty acids from adipose storage. What purpose does the increase in LPLA after exercise in fit subjects serve? Savard et al.[40] found a positive correlation between total work output and changes in subcutaneous AT LPLA. They speculated that AT LPLA may contribute to the supply of free fatty acid (FFA) to the muscle during exercise. How might this occur? Olivecrona and colleagues[43,44] suggested that increased LPLA contributes to an intracellular adipocyte pool of FFAs and, consequently, to an enhancement of their mobilization. Regardless of the tissue site of capillary endothelium-bound LPL, hydrolysis of circulating triglycerides releases fatty acids into the circulation.[45]

Studies of acute exercise in sedentary, overweight subjects are absent from the literature. It is doubtful that the results observed in lean, fit subjects generalize to the sedentary, overweight population. Only endurance-trained people can sustain long bouts of endurance exercise at high absolute and relative intensity levels. Furthermore, only lean individuals have small adipocytes. It may be that endurance exercise stimulates a rise in AT LPL only when cells are undersized.

### 3.4.2   Resistance exercise

Resistance exercise requires less total fuel and fat than endurance exercise. On this basis, LPL expression is not expected and human studies, thus, are not found. One study of rats compared two eating patterns that were scheduled around regular resistance exercise:[46] eating immediately vs. 4 hr after resistance training. Adipose tissue mass (perirenal, epididymal, and mesenteric) was 24% lower in rats that ate just after exercise, while muscle mass was 6% higher. Circulating insulin normally falls acutely with, but recovers hours after, resistance exercise. This fall may lower AT LPLA, perhaps impairing adipose tissue uptake of dietary triglyceride-derived fatty acids just after exercise.

## 3.5   Chronic endurance-training effect

In rats, some evidence shows a decrease (23 to 75%) in epididymal or retroperitoneal AT LPLA lasting up to 24 hr following exercise.[32,47] For example, Applegate et al.[47,48] found that treadmill running for 50 min/day, at 20 m/min for 6 weeks, decreased AT LPLTA at 24 hr post-exercise by 33% in epididymal[47] and 54 to 63% in retroperitoneal fat[47,48] of the male Osborne–Mendel rat. Other studies have shown relatively little effect of endurance training on adipose tissue LPL mRNA,[49] mass,[49] or activity.[34,49,50] It is noteworthy that training of obese Zucker rats further increased the already elevated AT LPLA in these animals.[50]

Studies in humans are relatively few. In 20 inactive, middle-aged (31 to 49 years old) men, Peltonen et al.[51] found that 15 weeks of training, with three bouts per week at a heart rate of 140 to 160 bpm for 30 to 60 min per bout, significantly increased subcutaneous abdominal AT LPLA by 56%, while a parallel control group increased nonsignificantly by 28%. Timing of the tissue samples was consistent within, but not across, subjects. Neither fat cell size nor body fat was measured; however, the men averaged 103% of ideal body weight for height.

Stubbe et al.[52] exercise-trained a similar group of men (mean percent body fat [%BF] = 28%; VO$_2$max = 33 to 36 mL O$_2$ kg$^{-1}$ min$^{-1}$) for 6 weeks at either moderate (68% of VO$_2$max) or high intensity (85% of VO$_2$max). Subcutaneous gluteal adipose tissue samples were taken pre- and post-training, presumably in the fasted state, 48 to 72 hr post-exercise. Adipose tissue HR-LPLA rose significantly by 50% post-training, while HDL-C rose by 7% when the groups were combined. The elevation of HDL-C was significantly related ($r = 0.50$) to the increase in AT HR-LPLA. In another study of healthy men (mean %BF = 19.6%; VO$_2$max = 40.6 mL O$_2$ kg$^{-1}$ min$^{-1}$), virtually no changes in subcutaneous thigh AT EXT-LPLA, HR-LPLA, LPL mRNA, or LPL mass occurred after short-term training consisting of 5 to 13 successive days at 65% of VO$_2$max, requiring 400 to 900 kcal per bout.[17] Samples were obtained 14 to 18 hr post-exercise in the fasted state. The workload was chosen to maximize the fat oxidation rate.[53] Plasma triglycerides fell 26% and HDL-C rose 4%, indicating metabolic training effects. Adipocyte size was not measured. In this study, the change in fasting triglycerides could not be predicted by the change in AT HR-LPLA, but the change was significantly related to the rise in skeletal muscle LPLA ($r = -0.45$).[17]

These studies of men show that increases in AT LPLA with training are modest. It is not clear whether lower fitness level, lesser exercise volume and/or intensity, higher body fat, different sampling time post-exercise, or site of adipose tissue sampling explains the lower response compared to acute bouts in endurance athletes.

Cessation of exercise training for 2 weeks in men and women accustomed to running >32 km/wk was studied by Simsolo et al.[23] In the trained state, subcutaneous abdominal tissue samples were taken one day after exercise. In both the trained and detrained condition, subjects were fasted for 12 hr. Based on acute and chronic exercise data, AT LPLA might be expected to decrease; however, subcutaneous abdominal LPL mRNA, total mass, and LPLTA did not change, and adipose tissue HR-LPLA and HR-LPL mass (both of which represented less than 10% of total activity and mass, respectively) increased significantly by 85 to 100%. The authors concluded that exercise regulates AT LPL post-translationally. Interestingly, the ratio of adipose to skeletal muscle LPLTA increased tenfold, from 0.51 ± 0.17 to 4.45 ± 2.46, with detraining. The changed ratio is evidence of the role of LPL in directing triglyceride-derived fatty acids to muscle during training and toward adipocyte storage when not exercise training.

## 3.5.1   Endurance training in overweight subjects

Lamarche et al.[54] studied obese (mean BMI = 34.1; %BF = 46%) premenopausal women (ages 35 ± 5 yr) before and after a 6-month endurance exercise training program of 90-min sessions 4 to 5 times per week at 50 to 55% of $VO_2max$ (i.e., low-intensity). Tissues were sampled in the early follicular phase of the menstrual cycle and in the post-training condition 24 to 48 hr after the last exercise bout. Abdominal and femoral AT HR-LPLA fell 55% and 35%, respectively, whether expressed per cell mass or surface area. Body mass tended to decrease by 1.5 kg, but this was not statistically significant. Mean adipocyte mass averaged $0.84 \pm 0.24$ and $0.91 \pm 0.18$ μg at the abdominal and femoral sites, respectively, and tended to decrease by about 10% with training. The fall in abdominal (but not femoral) AT HR-LPLA was significantly related to the decrease (32%) in the insulin/glucose area ratio following oral glucose challenge. Despite the fall in subcutaneous adipose tissue LPLA, exercise training raised post-heparin plasma lipase activity by >80%, consistent with the possibility that skeletal muscle LPLA increased.

Nicklas et al.[55] studied responses in 36 obese (body mass = $86.6 \pm 1.7$ kg; BMI = $33 \pm 0.6$; body fat = 51%) women. They enrolled in a 6-month weight-loss program in which energy restriction (250 to 300 kcal/day) and exercise (30 to 45 min/day at 50–60% of heart rate reserve) were combined. Fat mass loss was 5.9 kg, lean mass gain was 0.2 kg, and $VO_2max$ increased by 0.1 L $O_2$ $min^{-1}$ (6.1%, $p < 0.05$). Tissues were sampled after a 12-hr fast. Neither abdominal nor gluteal subcutaneous AT HR-LPLA changed, although trends toward a decrease at the abdominal site and an increase at the gluteal site were observed. Fat cell size was large (0.85 to 0.90 μg) and fell significantly to 0.74 to 0.79 μg post-training. Small, but significant, metabolic improvements occurred, including declines in fasting glucose, plasma total cholesterol, and triglycerides. A comparison of subjects who decreased vs. increased AT LPLA revealed that women who lowered AT LPLA with weight loss lowered both plasma total and low-density lipo-protein (LDL) cholesterol.

### 3.5.2 Hypothesis proposed by Lamarche et al.

The exercise effects on AT LPL in overweight subjects do not agree with those in lean, fit subjects. Lamarche et al.[54] attempted to unify these disparate findings. They proposed a U-shaped relationship between the level of basal subcutaneous AT LPLA and four categories of subjects that included: (1) obese and sedentary, (2) sedentary but not obese, (3) trained, and (4) very lean and highly trained. They further proposed that insulin responsiveness is low in category 1 subjects (obese and sedentary), becoming progressively greater in categories 2, 3, and 4.

### 3.5.3 Weight regain with detraining

The energy required for chronic endurance training can deplete adipose triglycerides. In rats, endurance exercise in large volumes can prevent fat mass gain, at least in part through suppression of AT LPLA.[56] Two studies show that detraining of rats restores LPLA within a week. Applegate and

Stern[47] found that 6 weeks of treadmill running at 20 m/min for 50 min/day decreased AT LPLTA at 24 hr post-exercise by 63% in the retroperitoneal fat, but only by 33% in epididymal fat. Detraining led to recovery of AT LPLTA between 48 and 60 hr in both depots. Recovery of AT LPLA to sedentary levels (after a threefold training-induced decrease) occurs within 1 week and contributes to weight regain after fat loss associated with endurance training.[33]

Rats that are calorie restricted and then re-fed experience a parallel loss and regain of body mass. At the end of two weight-loss/weight-regain cycles in rats fed a high-fat (45%) diet, LPL and the lipogenic enzymes fatty acid synthase, acetyl-CoA carboxylase, malic enzyme, and pyruvate kinase yielded an overshoot of activities.[57] These changes were accompanied by an 80% increase in the size of the adipocyte and a 40 to 50% increase in the size of perirenal and epididymal fat tissues.

In the months following weight loss, people often regain weight. The data of Nicklas et al.[55] suggest that the AT LPLA response during the weight-loss period influences subsequent weight change. Those who lowered AT LPLA more during exercise training tended to keep the weight off during 6 months of follow-up.

## 3.6   Mechanisms: hormones and intracellular factors

Lipoprotein lipase regulation *in vivo* is exceedingly complex, making a concise summary difficult. A number of hormones, especially insulin, play a role.

### 3.6.1   Insulin

Insulin promotes energy storage, a role affected in part by increasing adipose tissue LPLA. In the rat, tissue culture[58] and whole animal evidence[59] suggests that insulin in physiologic doses increases adipocyte LPL mRNA, indicating transcriptional regulation. Insulin in cultured adipocytes also increases LPL mRNA stability, allowing LPLA to increase without increased LPL gene transcription.[60] In non-obese human subcutaneous abdominal adipose tissue fragments maintained in organ culture, a supraphysiologic dose of insulin (10 nM) raised AT HR-LPLA and LPLTA by sevenfold, mostly through a fivefold increase in the LPL synthetic rate of LPL.[61] However, physiologic insulin does not increase human adipocyte LPL.[62-64] Thus, while adipose tissue LPLA correlates with serum insulin levels and the degree of insulin sensitivity under many circumstances,[22,65-68] it does not appear that insulin regulates LPL at the gene level.

### 3.6.2   Estrogen

Physiological estrogen may exert a tonic influence over the synthesis and ultimate destination of fatty acids. Wilson et al.[69] measured adipose tissue, heart, and diaphragm muscle LPLA in Sprague–Dawley rats after estrogen therapy of 5 µg/wk or 500 µg/wk. Samples were taken between 7 and 9 a.m. from fed animals. AT LPLA decreased by 75% and 95%, respectively, in response to estrogen therapy, while heart and diaphragm muscle LPLA increased by 110% and 140%. Fat tissue LPLA responses to fasting and re-feeding were blunted. Testosterone had no effect on any tissue. The results suggest that estrogen may shift the flux of triglyceride fatty acids from storage in the adipose organ toward incorporation by muscle.

## 3.6.3   Catecholamines

Epinephrine rises during high-intensity exercise and is a potential regulator of AT LPLA *in vivo*. Epinephrine decreased LPL translation and synthesis in mouse 3T3-L1 adipocytes via a *trans*-acting factor that binds to the 3′ untranslated region of LPL mRNA.[70] In normal rat adipocytes, the adrenergic agonist isoproterenol decreased LPL transcription within 15 min.[60] When injected into rats, norepinephrine raised LPL mRNA by 100 in intrascapular brown adipose tissue.[59] Finally, adrenalectomy reduced adiposity (and adipocyte size by 30%) of Sprague–Dawley rats fed standard chow; however, no effect on AT HR-LPLA was observed, and only a small increase in EXT-LPLA occurred. Cell size decreased, accounting for the increase in EXT-LPLA.[71]

## 3.6.4   Other hormones and factors

### 3.6.4.1   Growth hormone
Growth hormone stimulates a rise in LPL as preadipocytes differentiate into mature adipocytes. Barcellini-Couget et al.[105] showed that calcium abolishes the growth-hormone-stimulated rise in LPL seen in Ob1771 preadipose cells.

### 3.6.4.2   Thyroid hormone
Compared to controls, the epididymal fat pads of hypothyroid rats express a 4.5-fold higher HR-LPLA and threefold higher LPL mass due to an increased LPL synthetic rate.[73] As summarized by Bjorntorp,[9] cortisol and insulin together promote intra-abdominal adipocyte LPLA and promote lipid accumulation there. Tissue culture studies show that cortisol increases AT LPLA but requires insulin for its action. Ottosson et al.[75] showed that cortisol (1000 nmol/L) in the presence of insulin (7175 pmol/L) stimulated a 2.5-fold increase in LPL mRNA, a threefold increase in LPL synthesis, and a 9.4-fold increase in HR-LPLA. They concluded that cortisol regulated adipose LPL via both transcriptional regulation and additional post-translational regulation. In non-obese human subcutaneous abdominal adipose tissue fragments maintained in organ culture, dexamethasone (synthetic cortisol) increased AT HR-LPLA eightfold through inhibition of LPL degradation.[76]

### 3.6.4.3   Progesterone

Progesterone promotes filling of gluteo-femoral adipocytes by stimulating LPLA in these cells.[77]

### 3.6.4.4   Testosterone

Testosterone administered to men inhibits subcutaneous abdominal LPL but not femoral LPL.[78]

### 3.6.4.5   Tumor necrosis factor-alpha (TNF-α)

Kern et al.[79] postulated that TNF-α might regulate AT LPL. In human adipocytes taken from different subjects, those with the highest LPLTA (mean = 2.5-fold higher than others) had the lowest TNF-α. However, Kern et al.[79] concluded that TNF-α was not a main regulator of AT LPL because of a relatively weak correlation ($r = -0.39$) between TNF-α and LPL mRNA. Because serum TNF-α is elevated in Type II diabetes mellitus,[80] it is possible that AT LPL may be reduced or respond differently to exercise in diabetics.[52]

### 3.6.4.6   Leptin

Plasma leptin was found to be related to abdominal and gluteal AT HR-LPLA in older men who varied in both fitness and percent body fat.[28] The correlation was approximately 0.6, which was higher than that for insulin.

## 3.7   Non-exercise factors that affect the adipose tissue lipoprotein lipase response to exercise

### 3.7.1   Eating

In humans, eating acutely raises AT HR-LPLA and fasting lowers it. The changes are comparable in magnitude to exercise changes. For example, in fit, older men, subcutaneous abdominal and gluteal AT HR-LPLA rose 57% 4 hr postprandially.[81] The clearance of postprandial triglycerides is moderately related to AT HR-LPLA ($r = 0.42$).[81] It is interesting that the normal rise in AT HR-LPLA was absent in men who were insulin resistant.[81] Extended fasting lowers subcutaneous HR-LPLA by about 40%.[82] The changes in HR-LPLA and adipose tissue lipolytic activities, from baseline (overnight fast) to 7 days of fasting, are strongly and inversely related ($r = -0.81$ to $-0.85$),[82] emphasizing the reciprocal regulation of LPL and intracellular lipolysis.

In rats, feeding opposes exercise effects on AT LPLA. LPLTA shows a 24-hr diurnal pattern related to nocturnal eating.[83] LPL mass and LPLTA rise and fall together, peaking 8 hr after eating, while LPL mRNA in fed rats does not change.[83] Thus, regulation of the LPL response to eating is post-transcriptional, and an increase in inactive, monomeric lipase is evidence that regulation may be post-translational.[84]

In rats, during extended fasting, AT LPL rises due to transcriptional regulation. Fasting for 12 to 24 hr in the rat decreases AT LPLTA by 70% and LPL mass by 20 to 40%,[83] unrelated to LPL mRNA levels (which fall then rise). Compared to the fed state, extension of fasting to 36 hr reduces LPL mRNA by 50%; to 72 hr, by 70%.[83] LPLTA and mass both fall during fasting. In agreement, LaDu et al.[85] reported that 24 hr of fasting reduced rat AT LPLA by 59% and relative LPL mRNA concentrations by 25%. No long-term fasting LPL mRNA data exist for humans.

Ong et al.[49] examined the interactive effects of exercise training and eating in male Sprague–Dawley rats. Training was 90 to 120 min/day, 6 days/wk, for 6 weeks at a treadmill velocity of 25 m/min and 8% incline. Compared to control rats, body mass was 8% less and epididymal fat pad mass was 25% less. The results, summarized below, show that feeding has a stronger effect than acute or chronic exercise on AT LPL.

1. *Feeding vs. fasting without training:* Untrained, fed animals had higher epididymal fat HR-LPLA by 800%, HR-LPL mass by 100%, and EXT-LPLA by 100%, compared with untrained animals fasted for 17 to 19 hr.[49] These findings agree with the data of LaDu et al.[85] who found 24 hr of fasting reduced AT LPLA by 59% and relative LPL mRNA concentrations by 25%. EXT-LPL mass did not differ, nor did LPL mRNA, between fed and fasted rats.[49]

2. *Feeding vs. fasting in trained animals:* In trained rats, feeding induced changes slightly greater than those seen in untrained rats. Compared to trained, rested, and fasted rats, feeding increased HR-LPLA 1000%; HR-LPL mass, 120%; EXT-LPLA, 200%; and EXT-LPL mass, 70%. LPL mRNA was unaffected.

3. *Feeding response in trained vs. untrained:* When exercise-trained and fed animals were compared with controls, fed animals, differences again were small. HR-LPLA and mass were 26% and 70% higher, respectively, in the trained rats; EXT-LPLA was not different, but EXT-LPL mass was 24% higher.

In summary, exercise training (followed by 24 hr of rest) did not change the subsequent responses to (1) normal feeding or (2) 17 to 19 hr of fasting. Thus, in the rat, feeding, not exercise training, predominantly regulates AT LPL.

## 3.7.2    Other factors

### 3.7.2.1    Training state and fitness level

Because endurance athletes have low body fat, are aerobically fit, and have been reported to have high AT LPLA, it was not clear until recently whether fitness per se affected LPLA. However, Berman et al.[28] showed that leanness and adipocyte mass were more important than fitness level as a determinant of AT LPLA.

### 3.7.2.2   Gender

At rest, women's subcutaneous AT HR-LPLA per gram exceeds that of men by up to 500%.[24,86,87] Among the morbidly obese, subcutaneous LPLA is higher in women than in men.[88] The higher LPLA may help explain higher body fat in women than in men. Does gender affect the exercise LPL response? Faced with chronic exercise (3 to 18 months), healthy women defend fat mass more effectively than men.[89–91] None of these studies measured LPLA. Whether lipogenic enzymes increase or lipolytic enzymes are reduced is not yet clear. Despres et al.[89] showed that, after training, women had less suprailiac fat lipolytic response to epinephrine than men, but only men lost significant fat mass and decreased fat cell size.

### 3.7.2.3   Pregnancy

The tendency to increase internal body fat during pregnancy in rats is not due to increased LPLA, even though adipocyte size increases.[92] Swimming 3 hr per day, 6 days a week, throughout pregnancy in lean Zucker (Fa/Fa) rats prevented 20% of the normal weight gain.[56] Abdominal retroperitoneal and parametrial fat depots showed smaller and fewer adipocytes. Total LPLA in these tissues were suppressed compared to control pregnant rats, indicating that exercise decreased fat mass at least in part through lower LPLA.[56]

### 3.7.2.4   Regional site

Several animal studies have reported site-specific LPL responses to exercise. Savard et al.[93] swim-trained Zucker virgin, lean female homozygotes (Fa/Fa) for 5 weeks. Training was increased 15 min per day until, within 2 weeks, rats swam continuously for 3 hr. Adipose tissue samples were obtained 48 hr post-exercise at 14, 24, and 36 days of training. By 24 days, AT LPLTA had decreased 45 to 65% in retroperitoneal and parametrial fat pads, but had increased in the inguinal fat pad. At day 24, cell size decreased significantly in both deep sites. By day 36, LPLA rebounded to control levels in parametrial and near-control levels in retroperitoneal AT. The authors concluded that inguinal LPLA is not inhibited by exercise and that the rebound in deep-site LPLA represented preservation of a minimal adiposity. Applegate and Stern[47] found that 6 weeks of 50 min/day treadmill running, at 20 m/min, decreased AT LPLTA at 24 hr post-exercise by 63% in the retroperitoneal fat, but only by 33% in epididymal fat. Detraining led to recovery of AT LPLTA in both depots between 48 and 60 hr.

Pond et al.[94] examined AT LPLTA responses from nine different adipose tissue depots in untrained, 18-hr-fasted guinea pigs that exercised acutely for 30 min to near exhaustion just before sacrifice. Exercise decreased LPLTA in superficial intermuscular depots (35 to 41%) and in other superficial depots (around the forelimb and shoulder; interscapular) by 18 to 28%, but not in the dorsal wall of the abdomen, the groin, or fat around the heart.[94]

Fasting subcutaneous gluteal AT HR-LPLA is higher than abdominal in women, but in men subcutaneous abdominal LPL mRNA is about threefold higher than gluteal.[86] Mauriege et al.[29] reported lower subcutaneous abdominal AT HR-LPLA than femoral in both sedentary and trained women. In women, gluteal and femoral AT-LPLA is higher than abdominal in both obese[88] and normal-weight populations,[95] while in obese men, little variation in LPLA by region is observed.[88] In premenopausal, sedentary women who varied in %BF (range = 20 to 55%), subcutaneous femoral HR-LPLA was 50% higher than abdominal, and femoral fat cell weight was 22% larger.[96] In every case, correlations between abdominal LPLA and fatness were significant, but no relationship between femoral LPLA and body fat was found. In addition, correlations were high ($r$ = 0.68–0.82) between LPLA and adipocyte size (weight). Rebuffe-Scrive et al.[97,98] investigated differences between intra-abdominal and subcutaneous AT LPLA. They found that obese men had two- to threefold greater intra-abdominal AT LPLTA than their normal-weight counterparts, and obese women had four- to fivefold higher AT LPLTA than thin women. Among thin subjects, the men had larger intra-abdominal adipocytes than women, but lesser LPLA. In obese subjects, the adipocyte size was equally large in both sexes.

### 3.7.2.5 Adipocyte size

In lean, healthy persons without insulin resistance, AT HR-LPLA correlates with cell size.[41] In the study reported by Savard et al.,[41] mean cell weight ranged from 0.12 to 0.66 μg and HR-LPLA ranged from 0.13 to 0.74 μmol FFA hr$^{-1}$ 10$^6$ cells$^{-1}$, yielding a Pearson correlation of 0.80. Nevertheless, in obese adults, adipocytes are large with high LPLA. High LPLA may be due to increased post-translational activation by insulin[13] or perhaps abnormal regulation. During caloric restriction and weight loss, AT LPL activity declines;[101] however, transcriptional regulation helps raise AT LPLA during weight stabilization following weight loss.[102] An isocaloric mixed diet for one day after a 30% weight loss (42 kg) in very obese persons (mean BMI = 43) significantly raised subcutaneous abdominal AT HR-LPLA by 87%; EXT LPLA, 19%; HR LPL mass, 287%; EXT LPL mass, 73%; and LPL mRNA, 100%.[102] The LPL activity and mass increases were strongly related to initial BMI (Pearson $r$ = 0.8–0.9). Kern et al.[102] concluded that the increase in AT LPLA makes maintenance of weight loss difficult for the extremely obese, but this problem is minimal for those with BMI < 35 before weight loss.

### 3.7.2.6 Genotype

The subcutaneous suprailiac AT HR-LPLA response to 90 min of exercise (intensity at finish = 88% of max HR) was studied in monozygotic and dizygotic twin pairs. The within-pair rise was more closely related in monozygotic compared to dizygotic twins (intraclass $r$ = 0.87 vs. $r$ = 0.51).[41]

This suggests a genetic component to the response. Understanding this genetic component is a current challenge. Recently, Nicklas et al.[103] showed that subcutaneous AT HR-LPLA varied in relation to a common DNA polymorphism: the presence or complete absence of the cut-site for the restriction enzyme *PvuII* located in intron 6 of the LPL gene. Adipose tissue HR-LPLA decreased with the number of affected (+) *PvuII* alleles; it was highest in the (−/−) subjects, 36 to 39% lower in the (−/+) group, and 60% lower in the (+/+) group. In the (−/−) compared to the other two groups, fasting plasma total and LDL cholesterol levels were lower, but triglycerides did not differ. Why are there differences between groups when the protein product is identical? The authors proposed that the LPL *PvuII* cut-site is in linkage disequilibrium with one or more nearby functional mutations. It will be interesting to learn if this polymorphism affects the exercise response.

## 3.8 Tissue lipoprotein lipase and circulating lipoprotein lipid concentrations

Nikkila et al.[24] showed a very high correlation between fasting serum HDL cholesterol concentration and gluteal AT-LPLA in 52 normolipemic subjects ($r = 0.94$), but these findings have not been replicated. The opposite was found in fasting older men: abdominal AT HR-LPLA was negatively related ($r = -0.32$) and gluteal AT HR-LPLA was unrelated to plasma HDL-C.[28] In premenopausal women, Pouliot et al.[96] found that femoral AT HR-LPLA, but not abdominal, was significantly and positively related to HDL-C ($r = 0.4–0.5$). In postmenopausal women, femoral AT-LPLA and HDL$_2$-C (a subfraction of HDL-C) were positively related ($r = 0.69$).[87]

Whether or not a relationship is seen between adipose tissue LPLA or skeletal muscle LPLA and circulating lipids may depend on the timing of the tissue samples. This fact highlights the importance of tissue blood flow, total body adipose mass relative to body size, and food intake status. For a discussion of the relationship of skeletal muscle and adipose tissue LPL, see the review by Seip and Semenkovich.[104]

## 3.9 Summary

The effect of exercise on adipose tissue LPL is considerably less than that of feeding and fasting. Because of the modest effect of exercise, results have been confusing. In highly trained endurance athletes and in trained human subjects, acute exercise raises subcutaneous AT LPLA, although recent studies that have differed from the earlier studies in timing of tissue sampling dispute this. Acute exercise raises subcutaneous AT HR-LPLA by about 50% in trained persons performing long vigorous bouts; however, some of these results are confounded due to concomitant eating effects.

Two studies show that endurance training of humans increases subcutaneous LPLA,[51,52] but two others show no difference in LPLA,[23,55] and one study of endurance exercise training shows a decrease in LPLA.[54] In contrast to humans, exercise in rats tends to decrease AT LPLA. One fundamental difference between the animal and human studies is that animal studies have investigated internally deposited fat, which may respond differently than subcutaneous fat. An interesting model to explain different responses in thin and obese humans was put forth by Lamarche et al.,[54] who proposed that the adipocytes of obese subjects have higher basal LPLA and are therefore less responsive to exercise effects than adipocytes of lean, fit subjects. This model, however, does not fully explain the reported fall in AT LPLA with training in obese subjects. It is possible that other factors innate to the cells themselves determine the response to exercise. Finally, the response to exercise has a genetic component, as indicated by studies of mono- and dizygotic twins. Investigation to understand the nature of this component is just beginning.

## References

1. Olivecrona, T. and Bengtsson-Olivecrona, G., Lipoprotein lipase and hepatic lipase, *Curr. Opin. Lipid.*, 1, 222–230, 1990.
2. Storlien, L.H., Jenkins, A.B., Chisholm, D.J., Pascoe, W.S., Khouri, S., and Kraegen, E.W., Influence of dietary fat composition on development of insulin resistance in rats, *Diabetologia*, 40, 280–289, 1991.
3. Coleman, T., Seip, R.L., Gimble, J.M., Lee, D., Maeda, N., and Semenkovich, C.F., COOH-terminal disruption of lipoprotein lipase in mice is lethal in homozygotes, but heterozygotes have elevated triglycerides and impaired enzyme activity, *J. Biol. Chem.*, 270, 12518–12525, 1995.
4. Taskinen, M.-R., Nikkila, E.A., Huttunen, J.K., and Hilden, H., A micromethod for assay of lipoprotein lipase activity in needle biopsy samples of human adipose tissue and skeletal muscle, *Clinica Chimica Acta*, 104, 107–117, 1980.
5. Sady, S.P., Thompson, P.D., Cullinance, E.M., Kantor, M.A., Domagala, E., and Herbert, P.N., Prolonged exercise augments plasma triglyceride clearance, *JAMA*, 256, 2552–2555, 1986.
6. Goldberg, I.J., Lipoprotein lipase and lipolysis: central roles in lipoprotein metabolism and atherogenesis, *J. Lipid Res.*, 37, 693–707, 1996.
7. Miesenbock, G. and Patsch, J.R., Postprandial hyperlipemia: the search for the atherogenic protein, *Curr. Opin. Lipidol.*, 3, 196–201, 1992.
8. Gianturco, S.H. and Bradley, W.A., Pathophysiology of triglyceride-rich lipoproteins in atherothrombosis: cellular aspects, *Clin. Cardiol.*, 22(6, suppl.), II7–II14, 1999.
9. Bjorntorp, P., The regulation of adipose tissue distribution in man, *Int. J. Obesity* Relat. *Metab. Disord.*, 20, 291–302, 1996.
10. Neufer, P.D. and Dohm, G.L., Exercise induces a transient increase in transcription of the GLUT-4 gene in skeletal muscle, *Am. J. Physiol.*, 265, C1597–C1603, 1993.

11. Gyntelberg, F., Brennan, R., Holloszy, J.O., Schonfeld, G., Rennie, M.J., and Weidman, S.W., Plasma triglyceride lowering by exercise despite increased food intake in patients with type IV hyperlipoproteinemia, *Am. J. Clin. Nutr.*, 30, 716–720, 1977.

12. Seip, R.L., Mair, K., Cole, T.G., and Semenkovich, C.F., Induction of human skeletal muscle lipoprotein lipase gene expression by short-term exercise is transient, *Am. J. Physiol.*, 272, E255–E261, 1997.

13. Ong, J.M. and Kern, P.A., The role of glucose and glycosylation in the regulation of lipoprotein lipase synthesis and secretion in rat adipocytes, *J. Biol. Chem.*, 264, 3177–3182, 1989.

14. Frayn, K.N., Macronutrient metabolism of adipose tissue at rest and during exercise: a methodological viewpoint, *Proc. Nutr. Soc.*, 877–886, 2001.

15. Mulla, N.A.L., Simonsen, L., and Bülow, J., Post-exercise adipose tissue and skeletal muscle lipid metabolism in humans: the effect of exercise intensity, *J. Physiol.*, 524, 919–928, 2000.

16. Bulow, J., Adipose tissue blood flow during exercise, *Danish Med. Bull.*, 30, 85–100, 1983.

17. Seip, R.L., Angelopoulos, T.J., and Semenkovich, C.F., Exercise induces human lipoprotein lipase gene expression in skeletal muscle but not adipose tissue, *Am. J. Physiol.*, 268, E229–E236, 1995.

18. Borensztajn, J., Heart and skeletal muscle lipoprotein lipase, in *Lipoprotein Lipase*, J. Borensztajn, Ed., Evener, Chicago, 1987, pp. 133–148.

19. Lithell, H. and Boberg J., A method of determining lipoprotein-lipase activity in human adipose tissue, *Scand. J. Clin. Lab. Invest.*, 37, 551–561, 1977.

20. Iverius, P.-H. and Ostlund-Lindqvist, A.-M., Preparation, characterization, and measurement of lipoprotein lipase, *Meth. Enzymol.*, 129, 691–704, 1986.

21. Nilsson-Ehle, P., Measurements of lipoprotein lipase activity, in *Lipoprotein Lipase*, J. Borensztajn, Ed., Evener, Chicago, 1987, pp. 59–77.

22. Ong, J.M. and Kern, P.A., Effect of feeding and obesity on lipoprotein lipase activity, immunoreactive protein, and messenger RNA levels in human adipose tissue, *J. Clin. Invest.*, 84, 305–311, 1989.

23. Simsolo, R.B., Ong, J.M., and Kern, P.A., The regulation of adipose tissue and muscle lipoprotein lipase in runners by detraining, *J. Clin. Invest.*, 92, 2124–2130, 1993.

24. Nikkila, E.A., Taskinen, M.-R., Rehunen, S., and Harkonen, M., Lipoprotein lipase activity in adipose tissue and skeletal muscle of runners: relation to serum lipoproteins, *Metabolism*, 27, 1661–1671, 1978.

25. Marniemi, J., Peltonen, P., Vuori, I., and Hietanen, E., Lipoprotein lipase of human postheparin plasma and adipose tissue in relation to physical training, *Acta Physiol. Scand.*, 110, 131–135, 1980.

26. Peltonen, P., Marniemi, J., Vuori, I., and Hietanen, E., Physical training and lipoprotein lipase in man, *Biochem. Exer.*, 267–274, 1981.

27. Savard, R., Despres, J.-P., Marcotte, M., and Bouchard, C., Adipose tissue lipid accumulation pathways in marathon runners, *Int. J. Sports Med.*, 6, 287–291, 1985.

28. Berman, D.M., Rogus, E.M., Busby-Whitehead, M.J., Katzel, L.I., and Goldberg, A.P., Predictors of adipose tissue lipoprotein lipase in middle-aged and older men: relationship to leptin and obesity, but not cardiovascular fitness, *Metabolism*, 48, 183–189, 1999.

29. Mauriege, P., Prud'homme, D., Marcotte, M., Yoshioka, M., Tremblay, A., and Despres, J.P., Regional differences in adipose tissue metabolism between sedentary and endurance-trained women, *Am. J. Physiol.*, 273, E497–E506, 1997.

30. Nikkila, E.A., Torsti, P., and Penttila O., The effect of exercise on lipoprotein lipase activity of rat heart, adipose tissue and skeletal muscle, *Metabolism*, 12, 863–865, 1963.

31. Barakat, H.A., Kerr, D.S., Tapscott, E.B., and Dohm, G.L., Changes in plasma lipids and lipolytic activity during recovery from exercise of untrained rats, *Proc. Soc. Exp. Biol. Med.*, 166, 162–166, 1981.

32. Rauramaa, R., Acute effect of physical exercise on glycogen content and lipoprotein lipase activity in untrained diabetic rats, *Med. Biol.*, 60, 139–143, 1982.

33. Lambert, E.V., Wooding, G., Lambert, M.I., and Noakes, T.D., Enhanced adipose tissue lipoprotein lipase activity in detrained rats: independent of changes in food intake, *J. Appl. Physiol.*, 77, 2564–2571, 1994.

34. Askew, E.W., Dohm, G.L., Huston, R.L., Sneed, T.W., and Downall, H.J., Response of rat tissue lipases to physical training and exercise, *Proc. Soc. Exp. Biol. Med.*, 141, 123–129, 1972.

35. Eckel, R.H., Adipose tissue lipoprotein lipase, in *Lipoprotein Lipase*, J. Borensztajn, Ed., Evener, Chicago, 1988, pp. 79–132.

36. Paulin, A., Lalonde, J., and Deshaies, Y., Beta-adrenergic blockade and lipoprotein lipase activity in rat tissue after acute exercise, *Am. J. Physiol.*, 261, R891–R897, 1991.

37. Paulin, A. and Deshaies Y., Serum-free fatty acids are not involved in acute exercise-induced reduction of LPL in rat tissues, *Am. J. Physiol.*, 262, E377–E382, 1992.

38. LaDu, M.J., Kapsas, H., and Palmer, W.K., Regulation of lipoprotein lipase in adipose and muscle tissues during exercise, *J. Appl. Physiol.*, 71, 404–409, 1991.

39. Lithell, H., Hellsing, K., Lundqvist, G., and Malmberg, P., Lipoprotein-lipase activity of human skeletal-muscle and adipose tissue after intensive physical exercise, *Acta Physiol. Scand.*, 105, 312–315, 1979.

40. Savard, R., Despres, J.P., Marcotte, M., Theriault, G., Tremblay, A., and Bouchard, C., Acute effects of endurance exercise on human adipose tissue metabolism, *Metabolism*, 36(5), 480–485, 1987.

41. Savard, R. and Bouchard, C., Genetic effects in the response of adipose tissue lipoprotein lipase activity to prolonged exercise: a twin study, *Int. J. Obesity*, 14, 771–777, 1990.

42. Taskinen, M.R., Nikkila, E.A., Rehunen, S., and Gordin, A., Effect of acute vigorous exercise on lipoprotein lipase activity of adipose tissue and skeletal muscle in physically active men, *Artery*, 6(6), 471–483, 1980.

43. Ekstedt, B. and Olivecrona, T., Uptake and release of fatty acids by rat adipose tissue: last in to first out?, *Lipids*, 10, 858–860, 1970.

44. Olivecrona, T. and Bengtsson, G., Molecular basis for the interaction of lipoprotein lipase with triglyceride-rich lipoproteins at the capillary endothelium, in *Obesity: Cellular and Molecular Aspects*, G. Ailhaud, Ed., Inserm, Nice, France, 1979, pp. 125–136.

45. Scow, R.O., Hamosh, M., Blanchette-Mackie, E.J., and Evans, A.J., Uptake of blood triglyceride by various tissues, *Lipids*, 8, 497–505, 1972.

46. Suzuki, M., Doi, T., Okamura, K., Shimitsu, S., Okano, G., Sato, Y. et al., Effect of meal timing after resistance exercise on hindlimb muscle mass and fat accumulation in trained rats, *J. Nutr. Sci. Vitaminol. (Tokyo)*, 45, 401–409, 1999.

47. Applegate, E.A. and Stern, J.S., Exercise termination effects on food intake, plasma insulin, and adipose lipoprotein lipase activity in the Osborne–Mendel rat, *Metabolism*, 36, 709–714, 1987.

48. Applegate, E.A., Upton, D.E., and Stern, J.S., Exercise and detraining: effect on food intake, adiposity and lipogenesis in Osborne–Mendel rats made obese by a high-fat diet, *J. Nutr.*, 114, 447–459, 1984.

49. Ong, J.M., Simsolo, R.B., Saghizadeh, M., Goers, J.W., and Kern, P.A., Effects of exercise training and feeding on lipoprotein lipase gene expression in adipose tissue, heart, and skeletal muscle of the rat, *Metabolism*, 44(12), 1596–1605, 1995.

50. Walberg, J.L., Greenwood, M.R., and Stern, J.S., Lipoprotein lipase activity and lipolysis after swim training in obese Zucker rats, *Am. J. Physiol.*, 245, R706–R712, 1983.

51. Peltonen, P., Marniemi, J., Hietanen, E., Vuori, I., and Ehnholm, C., Changes in serum lipids, lipoproteins, and heparin-releasable lipolytic enzymes during moderate physical training in man: a longitudinal study, *Metabolism*, 30(5), 518–526, 1981.

52. Stubbe, I., Hansson, P., Gustafson, A., and Nilsson-Ehle, P., Plasma lipoproteins and lipolytic enzyme activites during endurance training in sedentary men: changes in high-density lipoprotein subfractions and composition, *Metabolism*, 32, 1120–1128, 1983.

53. Romijn, J.A., Coyle, E.F., Sidossis, S., Gastaldelli, A., Horowitz, J.F., Endert, E. et al. Regulation of endogenous fat and carbohydrate metabolism in relation to exercise intensity and duration, *Am. J. Physiol.*, 28, E380–E391, 1993.

54. Lamarche, B., Després, J.P., Moorjani, S., Nadeau, A., Lupien, P.-J., Tremblay, A. et al. Evidence for the role of insulin in the regulation of abdominal tissue lipoprotein lipase response to exercise training in obese women. *Int. J. Obesity*, 17, 255-261, 1993.

55. Nicklas, B.J., Rogus, E.M., Berman, D.M., Dennis, K.E., and Goldberg, A.P., Responses of adipose tissue lipoprotein lipase to weight loss affect lipid levels and weight regain in women, *Am. J. Physiol.*, 279, E1012–E1019, 2000.

56. Savard, R., Palmer, J.E., and Greenwood, M.R., Effects of exercise training on regional adipose tissue metabolism in pregnant rats, *Am. J. Physiol.*, 250, R837–R844, 1986.

57. Sea, M.M., Fong, W.P., Huang, Y., and Chen, Z.Y., Weight cycling-induced alteration in fatty acid metabolism, *Am. J. Physiol.*, 279, R1145–1155, 2000.

58. Ong, J.M., Kirchgessner, T.G., Schotz, M.C., and Kern, P.A., Insulin increases the synthetic rate and messenger RNA level of lipoprotein lipase in isolated rat adipocytes, *J. Biol. Chem.*, 263, 12933–12938, 1988.

59. Mitchell, J.R.D., Jacobsson, A., Kirchgessner, T.G., Schotz, M.C., Cannon, B., and Nedergaard, J., Regulation of expression of the lipoprotein lipase gene in brown adipose tissue, *Am. J. Physiol.*, 263, E500–E506, 1992.

60. Raynolds, M.V., Awald, P.D., Gordon, D.F., Gutiierrez-Hartmann, A., Rule, D.C., Wood, W.M. et al., Lipoprotein lipase gene expression in rat adipocytes is regulated by isoproterenol and insulin through different mechanisms, *Molec. Endocrinol.*, 4, 1416–1422, 1990.

61. Appel, B. and Fried, S.K., Effects of insulin and dexamethasone on lipoprotein lipase in human adipose tissue, *Endocrinol. Metab.*, 25, E695–E699, 1992.

62. Kern, P.A., Marshall, S., and Eckel, R.H., Regulation of lipoprotein lipase in primary cultures of isolated human adipocytes, *J. Clin. Invest.*, 75, 199–208, 1985.

63. Kern, P.A., Svoboda, M.E., Eckel, R.H., and Van Wyck, J.J., Insulin-like growth factor action and production in adipocytes and endothelial cells, *Diabetes*, 38, 710–717, 1989.

64. Kern, P.A., Ong, J.M., Goers, J.F., and Pedersen, M.E., Regulation of lipoprotein lipase immunoreactive mass in isolated human adiopcytes, *J. Clin. Invest.*, 81, 398–406, 1988.

65. Simsolo, R.B., Ong, J.M., Saffari, B., and Kern, P.A., Effect of improved diabetes control on the expression of lipoprotein lipase in human adipose tissue, *J. Lipid Res.*, 33, 89–95, 1992.

66. Pykalisto, O., Smith, P.H., and Brunzell, J.D. Determinants of human adipose tissue lipoprotein lipase. Effect of diabetes and obesity on basal- and diet-induced activity, *J. Clin. Invest.*, 56, 1108–1116, 1975.

67. Taskinen, M.-R. and Nikkila, E.A., Lipoprotein lipase activity of adipose tissue and skeletal muscle in insulin-deficient diabetes, *Diabetologia*, 17, 351–356, 1979.

68. Sadur, C.N. and Eckel, R.H., Insulin stimulation of adipose tissue lipoprotein lipase. Use of the euglycemic clamp technique, *J. Clin. Invest.*, 69, 1119–1125, 1982.

69. Wilson, D.E., Flowers, C.M., Carlile, S.I., and Udall, K.S., Estrogen treatment and gonadal function in the regulation of lipoprotein lipase, *Atherosclerosis*, 24, 491–499, 1976.

70. Yukht, A., Davis, R.C., Ong, J.M., Ranganathan, G., and Kern, P.A., Regulation of lipoprotein lipase translation by epinephrine in 3T3-L1 cells: importance of the 3' untranslated region, *J. Clin. Invest.*, 96, 2438–2444, 1995.

71. Edens, N.K., Moshirfar, A., Potter, G.M., Fried, S.K., and Castonguay, T.W., Adrenalectomy reduces adiposity by decreasing food efficiency, not direct effects on white adipose tissue, *Obesity Res.*, 7, 395–401, 1999.

72. Sambandam, N., Chen, X.S., Cam, M.C., and Rodrigues, B., Cardiac lipoprotein lipase in the spontaneously hypertensive rat, *Cardiovasc. Res.*, 33, 460–468, 1997.

73. Saffari, B., Ong, J.M., and Kern, P.A., Regulation of adipose tissue lipoprotein lipase gene expression by thyroid hormone in rats, *J. Lipid Res.*, 33, 241–249, 1992.

74. Rebuffe-Scrive, M., Krotkiewski, M., Elfverson, J., and Bjorntorp, P., Muscle and adipose tissue morphology and metabolism in Cushing's syndrome, *J. Clin. Endocrinol. Metab.*, 67, 1122–1128, 1988.

75. Ottosson, M., Vikman-Adolfsson, K., Enerback, S., Olivecrona, G., and Bjorntorp P., The effects of cortisol on the regulation of lipoprotein lipase activity in human adipose tissue, *J. Clin. Endocrinol. Metab.*, 79, 820–825, 1994.

76. Olefsky, J.M. and Nolan, J.J., Insulin resistance and non-insulin-dependent diabetes mellitus: cellular and molecular mechanisms, *Am. J. Clin. Nutr.*, 61(suppl.), 980S–986S, 1995.

77. Rebuffe-Scrive, M., Basdevant, A., and Guy-Grand, B., Effect of local application of progesterone on human adipose tissue lipoprotein lipase, *Horm. Metab. Res.*, 15, 566, 1985.

78. Rebuffe-Scrive, M., Marin, P., and Bjorntorp P., Effect of testosterone on abdominal adipose tissue in men, *Int. J. Obesity*, 15, 791–795, 1991.

79. Kern, P.A., Saghizadeh, M., Ong, J.M., Bosch, R.J., Deem, R., and Simsolo, R.B., The expression of tumor necrosis factor in human adipose tissue, *J. Clin. Invest.*, 95, 2111–2119, 1995.

80. Katsuki, A., Sumida, Y., Murashami, S., Murata, K., Takarada, Y., Ito, K.F.M. et al., Serum levels of tumor necrosis factor-alpha are increased in obese NIDDM patients, and levels are related to visceral fat, *J. Clin. Endocrinol. Metab.*, 83, 859–862, 1998.

81. Beltz, W.F., Kesaniemi, Y.A., Howard, B.V., and Grundy, S.M., Development of an integrated model for analysis of the kinetics of apolipoprotein B in plasma very low density lipoproteins, intermediate density lipoproteins, and low density lipoproteins, *J. Clin. Invest.*, 76, 575–585, 1985.

82. Arner, P., Bolinder, J., Engfeldt, P., and Lithell, H., The relationship between the basal lipolytic and lipoprotein lipase activities in human adipose tissue, *Int. J. Obesity*, 7, 167–172, 1983.

83. Bergo, M., Olivecrona, G., and Olivecrona, T., Diurnal rhythms and effects of fasting and refeeding on rat adipose tissue lipoprotein lipase, *Am. J. Physiol.*, 271, E1092–E1097, 1996.

84. Bergo, M., Olivecrona, G., and Olivecrona, T., Forms of lipoprotein lipase in rat tissues: in adipose tissue the proportion of inactive lipase increases on fasting, *Biochem. J.*, 313, 893–898, 1996.

85. LaDu, M.J., Kapsas, H., and Palmer, W.K., Regulation of lipoprotein lipase in adipose and muscle tissues during fasting, *Am. J. Physiol.*, 260, R953–R960, 1991.

86. Arner, P., Lithell, H., Wahrenberg, H., and Bronnegard, M., Expression of lipoprotein lipase in different human subcutaneous adipose tissue regions, *J. Lipid Res.*, 32, 423–428, 1991.

87. St.-Amand, J., Despres, J.-P., Lemieux, S., Lamarche, B., Moorjani, S., Prud'homme, D. et al., Does lipoprotein or hepatic lipase activity explain the protective lipoprotein profile of premenopausal women?, *Metabolism*, 44, 491–498, 1995.

88. Fried, S.K. and Kral, J.G., Sex differences in regional distribution of fat cell size and lipoprotein lipase activity in morbidly obese patients, *Int. J. Obesity*, 11, 129–140, 2001.

89. Despres, J.P., Bouchard, C., Savard, R., Tramblay, A., Marcotte, M., and Theriault, G., The effect of a 20-week endurance training program on adipose tissue morphology and lipolysis in men and women, *Metabolism*, 33, 235–239, 1984.

90. Andersson, B., Xu, X.F., Rebuffe-Scrive, M., Terning, K., Krotkiewski, M., and Bjorntorp, P., The effects of exercise training on body composition and metabolism in men and women, *Int. J. Obesity*, 15, 75–81, 1991.

91. Campbell, A.R., Jacobsen, D.J., and Donnelly, J.E., Effects of 16 months of exercise on visceral and subcutaneous fat in responders and non-responders [abstract], *Med. Sci. Sports Exerc.*, 32, S355–S355, 2000.

92. Sahlstrom, A., Petterson, U., and Forsum, E., Triglyceride turnover, lipoprotein lipase activity, and fat cell size in adipose tissue of rats during the first 2 weeks of pregnancy, *Ann. Nutr. Metab.*, 42, 55–62, 1998.

 93. Savard, R. and Greenwood, M.R., Site-specfic adipose tissue LPL responses to endurance training in female lean Zucker rats, *J. Appl. Physiol.*, 65, 693–699, 2001.
 94. Pond, C.M., Mattacks, C.A., and Sadler, D., The effects of exercise and feeding on the activity of lipoprotein lipase in nine different adipose depots of guinea pigs, *Int. J. Biochem.*, 24(11), 1825–1831, 1992.
 95. Rebuffe-Scrive, M., Enk, L., Crona, N., Lonnroth, P., Abrahamsson, L., and Bjorntorp, P., Fat cell metabolism in different regions in women. Effect of menstrual cycle, pregnancy, and lactation, *J. Clin. Invest.*, 75, 1973–1976, 1985.
 96. Pouliot, M.-C., Despres, J.-P., Moorjani, S., Lupien, P.J., Tremblay, A., Nadeau, A. et al., Regional variation in adipose tissue lipoprotein lipase activity: association with plasma high density lipoprotein levels, *Eur. J. Clin. Invest.*, 21, 398–405, 1991.
 97. Rebuffe-Scrive, M., Andersson, B., Olbe, L., and Bjorntorp, P., Metabolism of adipose tissue in intra-abdominal depots of nonobese men and women, *Metabolism*, 38, 453–458, 1989.
 98. Rebuffe-Scrive, M., Andersson, B., Olbe, L., and Bjorntorp, P., Metabolism of adipose tissue in intra-abdominal depots of severely obese men and women, *Metabolism*, 39, 1021–1025, 1990.
 99. Despres, J.P., Pouliot, M.C., Moorjani, S., Nadeau, A., Tremblay, A., Lupien, P.J. et al., Loss of abdominal fat and metabolic response to exercise training in obese women, *Am. J. Physiol.*, 261, E159–E167, 1991.
100. Schwartz, R.S., Cain, K.C., Shuman, W.C., Larson, V., Stratton, J.R., Beard, J.C. et al., Effect of intensive endurance training on lipoprotein profiles in young and older men, *Metabolism*, 41, 649–654, 1992.
101. Schwartz, R.S. and Brunzell, J.D., Increase of adipose tissue lipoprotein lipase activity with weight loss, *J. Clin. Invest.*, 67, 1425–1430, 1981.
102. Kern, P.A., Ong, J.M., Saffari, B., and Carty, J., The effects of weight loss on the activity and expression of adipose-tissue lipoprotein lipase in very obese humans, *New Engl. J. Med.*, 322, 1053–1059, 1990.
103. Nicklas, B., Ferrell, R.E., Rogus, E.M., Berman, D.M., Ryan, A.S., Dennis, K.E. et al., Lipoprotein lipase gene variation is associated with adipose tissue lipoprotein lipase activity, and lipoprotein lipid and glucose concentrations in overweight postmenopausal women, *Hum. Genet.*, 106, 420–424, 2000.
104. Seip, R.L. and Semenkovich, C.F., Skeletal muscle lipoprotein lipase: molecular regulation and physiological effects in relation to exercise, *Exercise Sports Sci. Rev.*, 26, 191–218, 1998.
105. Barcellini-Couget, S. et al., Rise in cytosolic $Ca^{2+}$ abolishes in preadipose cells the expression of lipoprotein lipase stimulated by growth hormone, *Biochem. Biophys. Res. Commun.*, 199(1), 136–143, 1994.

# chapter four

# Effects of acute endurance exercise and physical training on glucose metabolism in white adipose tissue

*Bente Stallknecht*

## Contents

## 4.1   Introduction

The influence of acute exercise and physical training on glucose metabolism in skeletal muscle has been examined extensively;[1-3] however, the influence of exercise and physical training on adipose tissue glucose metabolism has received far less attention. Most knowledge about adipose tissue metabolism in relation to exercise comes from *in vitro* studies that examine the effect of endurance training on lipolysis in adipocytes.[4,5] Nevertheless, a number of experiments that examine the effect of acute exercise and physical training on *in vitro* and *in vivo* glucose metabolism in rat and human adipose tissue have been performed. The roles of skeletal muscle and adipose tissue are different in relation to acute exercise. Skeletal muscle extracts lipids and glucose, which are used as energy during exercise,[1-3,6] whereas adipose tissue provides energy by lipolysis of stored triacylglycerol (TG).[6-8]

## 4.2   Adipose tissue glucose metabolism

Triacylglycerol stores in adipose tissue must be rebuilt between exercise sessions. TG is composed of three fatty acids that are esterified to a glycerol molecule.[9] After a meal, the fatty acids are supplied to the adipose tissue from the gut in the form of chylomicrons.[10-12] Furthermore, fatty acids are supplied to the adipose tissue in the form of lipoproteins, which are produced by the liver.[10-12] In addition, fatty acids can be synthesized from glucose in adipocytes, a process termed *de novo* lipogenesis (see Figure 4.1).[10,12] However, net lipogenesis is insignificant in humans on a typical Western diet.[10,12,13] Before esterification, fatty acids are activated by formation of a CoA-derivative, a process that requires adenosine triphosphate (ATP).[9] This ATP comes, at least partly, from oxidation of glucose in the adipocyte (Figure 4.1).[12,14] Glycerol, in itself, cannot be esterified to fatty acids and must be in its phosphorylated form (glycerol 3-phosphate) before esterification.[9,10] Glycerol 3-phosphate is formed in the adipocyte from glucose through glycolysis (Figure 4.1).[10] Glycerol 3-phosphate cannot be formed directly from glycerol to any significant degree in adipose tissue, as the activity of the enzyme catalyzing this process, glycerol kinase, is very low in adipose tissue.[15,16] Based on this analysis, it appears that glucose is a necessary metabolite for the formation of TG in adipocytes.

Adipocytes take up glucose,[10,14,17-19] and the glucose is transported, as in skeletal muscle, over the plasma membrane by a glucose transporter protein molecule (Figure 4.1).[20,21] In the adipocyte, glucose undergoes glycolysis, goes through the pentose phosphate pathway, or is stored as glycogen (Figure 4.1).[9] Through glycolysis, glucose is converted to glycerol 3-phosphate or fatty acids, metabolized to lactate, or oxidized to provide ATP for the adipocyte (Figure 4.1).[9] The pentose phosphate pathway produces NADPH (the reduced form of nicotinamide-adenine dinucleotide phosphate [NADP]), which is used during *de novo* lipogenesis (Figure 4.1).[9] Glycogen stores are low in adipose tissue but have been shown to increase after eating a high-carbohydrate diet.[22]

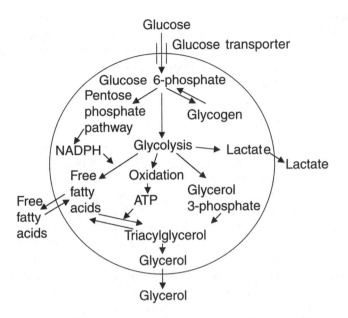

*Figure 4.1*   Schematic view of glucose metabolism in adipocytes.

Insulin and epinephrine are the two major hormones influencing adipose tissue metabolism.[10,12,17,23] Both insulin and epinephrine stimulate *in vitro* glucose transport in adipocytes[24-27] and *in vivo* glucose uptake in adipose tissue.[28-30] During exercise sessions, plasma epinephrine concentrations are increased and plasma insulin concentrations are decreased,[31] and between exercise sessions, especially after meals, plasma insulin concentrations are increased.[10,12,17] Accordingly, the change in adipose tissue glucose metabolism during and between exercise is difficult to predict from changes in hormone concentrations.

## 4.3   Methods for studying adipose tissue metabolism

Adipose tissue, especially from rats, has been studied extensively *in vitro*, but the tissue is difficult to study *in vivo*, especially in humans, because most depots do not have a vein that selectively drains the tissue and is easy to cannulate.[12] In the late 1980s, however, two new techniques for studying human adipose tissue metabolism *in vivo* emerged. Frayn and co-workers[32] developed a method for sampling the venous drainage from the subcutaneous adipose tissue of the anterior abdominal wall, and they have since evaluated many aspects of adipose tissue metabolism using the technique.[8,17,33] The vein cannulation, however, is difficult to perform, and it is difficult to draw blood from the vein because the blood flow in the vein is low. This is probably why only a few research groups have applied the technique. The other new *in vivo* technique for studying adipose tissue metabolism is the microdialysis technique, first applied by Lönnroth and co-workers[34] in human adipose tissue and by Arner and co-workers[35] in rat adipose tissue. Since then, microdialysis has been widely applied for studies of human and rat adipose tissue.[36–39] The abdominal vein catheterization and microdialysis techniques were compared, and it was concluded that the two techniques were complementary.[40]

## 4.4   Effect of acute exercise on glucose metabolism

The effect of acute exercise on glucose metabolism in adipose tissue is summarized here. Recently, the abdominal vein catheterization technique was used to estimate subcutaneous adipose tissue glucose uptake in young, healthy men during exercise on a cycle ergometer for 90 min at 40% of $VO_2$max or for 60 min at 60% of $VO_2$max.[41] Adipose tissue glucose uptake did not change in a statistically significant way during exercise or for 3 hr post-exercise in either exercise group.[41] Average adipose tissue glucose uptake, however, dropped from a pre-exercise value of approximately 0.7 $\mu$mol 100 $g^{-1}$ $min^{-1}$ to approximately 0.0 $\mu$mol 100 $g^{-1}$ $min^{-1}$ during the exercise, and rose during the post-exercise period again to approximately 0.7 $\mu$mol 100 $g^{-1}$ $min^{-1}$ in both groups.[41] The fact that the drop in glucose uptake during exercise was not significant could be due to the small arteriovenous difference for glucose across adipose tissue and the resulting variability in the calculated glucose uptake. However, in the same study, lactate output from adipose tissue increased significantly during exercise at 40% of $VO_2$max, indicating an increased glucose turnover at this exercise intensity.[41]

In 1987, two studies were published that examined the effect of cycle ergometer exercise on *in vitro* glucose metabolism in gluteal adipocytes from young, healthy men.[42,43] In the study by Koivisto et al.,[42] subjects cycled at a lower intensity and for a longer duration (45–50% of $VO_2$max for 3 hr) compared with the study by Savard et al.,[43] in which subjects maintained 88% of maximal heart rate for 90 min. In both studies, basal glucose metabolism (glucose transport[42] and glucose conversion to TG,[43] respectively) was decreased by exercise. Insulin binding to adipocytes was not altered by the exercise session,[42] but the percentage increase in glucose metabolism after insulin stimulation was increased by exercise in both studies.[42,43]

In rats, a single run to exhaustion immediately prior to sacrifice decreased *in vitro* insulin-stimulated glucose conversion to TG in epididymal adipose tissue of trained but not of sedentary rats.[44] Also, the activity of the enzyme-catalyzing TG synthesis (fatty acid synthetase) decreased after exercise in epididymal adipose tissue of trained but not of sedentary rats (when expressed per milligram of protein in adipose tissue homogenate).[44] To become exhausted, trained rats ran at a higher intensity for a longer duration compared with sedentary rats;[44] hence, the higher absolute workload performed by the trained rats, rather than a training-induced metabolic difference, might have reduced the TG synthesis of the trained rats.[44] Using the same experimental design, Askew et al.[45] examined the effect of exhaustive exercise on other enzymes involved in lipid synthesis in adipose tissue. The activities of ATP citrate-lyase, malic enzyme, and glyceride synthetase in epididymal adipose tissue were unchanged by exhaustive exercise, whereas the activity of glucose 6-phosphate dehydrogenase (from the pentose phosphate pathway) decreased with exercise in sedentary but not in trained rats.[45] The authors interpreted the decrease in glucose 6-phosphate dehydrogenase activity in sedentary rats as a shunting of glucose away from the pentose phosphate pathway so that glucose was available for more critical metabolic needs during exercise.[45] The lack of decrease in enzyme activity in trained rats was explained by the already lower glucose 6-phosphate dehydrogenase activity in trained compared with sedentary rats.[45]

A single swim to exhaustion 24 hr prior to sacrifice did not affect basal or insulin-stimulated glucose incorporation into TG in epididymal adipose tissue in sedentary rats.[46] Timing of sacrifice (rats) or fat biopsy (humans) after the exercise bout may greatly influence the effect of exercise found. The change with time after an acute exercise bout in adipose tissue glucose metabolism has not been examined systematically. However, whole-body, insulin-stimulated glucose uptake in rats does increase with time from 1 to 6 hours after an acute exercise bout, with no difference 6 and 24 hr post-exercise.[47]

In obese rats, 60 min of swimming followed by 60 min of rest increased basal and insulin-stimulated glucose transport rates (both at physiological and supraphysiological insulin concentrations) in epididymal adipocytes.[48] However, insulin sensitivity with regard to glucose transport in adipocytes was not affected.[48] Whether the difference between this study and other studies that have examined the effect of acute exercise on adipose tissue glucose metabolism is due to differences in experimental protocol (e.g., time after exercise, different aspects of glucose metabolism, the use of obese rats) is unknown. However, before exercise, the obese rats had decreased basal and maximally insulin-stimulated glucose transport rates compared with normal-weight rats,[48] and this might have influenced the response to exercise.

In conclusion, an acute bout of exercise appears to decrease basal and insulin-stimulated glucose transport and *de novo* lipogenesis in adipose tissue of normal-weight individuals, but further research is needed to confirm this.

## 4.5   Effect of physical training on glucose metabolism

Many studies have investigated the effect of physical training on glucose metabolism in adipose tissue. When examining the effect of physical training on adipose tissue metabolism it is important to take into account that physically trained individuals usually have a lower adipose tissue mass and smaller adipocytes compared with sedentary individuals.[49] The lower adipose tissue mass implies that differences in metabolism expressed per amount of adipose tissue (e.g., per 100 g of adipose tissue) do not necessarily reflect whole-body differences. The difference in adipocyte size between trained and sedentary individuals is important because adipocyte size per se influences adipocyte metabolism. Generally, basal and insulin-stimulated glucose metabolism expressed per adipocyte increases with adipocyte size in individuals of similar age.[50-53] Moreover, adipocyte glucose metabolism is more closely related to adipocyte surface area than to adipocyte weight or diameter,[51] implying that a way of normalizing for cell size is to express metabolism per adipocyte surface area. Unfortunately, most authors only express adipocyte metabolism data per adipocyte. Younger rats have smaller adipocytes compared with older rats, and in order to compare adipocytes from trained rats with adipocytes of similar size from sedentary rats, a younger control group has been included in some studies.[19,54-58] A complication in this approach is that, although adipocyte glucose metabolism increases with cell size per se, it also decreases with age,[52,53] and it is, accordingly, difficult to predict the difference in adipocyte glucose metabolism between rats of different age.

In the 1970s and early 1980s, most studies examining the effect of physical training on adipose tissue glucose metabolism were *in vitro* studies performed in rat adipocytes.[19,44,46,50,54-71] From the mid-1980s, studies were conducted in humans to examine the effect of physical training on *in vitro* glucose metabolism in adipocytes;[72-77] also, one *in vivo* study that examined the effect of training on glucose uptake in various tissues, including adipose tissue, was published.[78] Recently, more *in vivo* studies on the effect of training on glucose metabolism in adipose tissue were published.[28,79-81]

## 4.5.1   In vitro *glucose transport*

### 4.5.1.1   *Basal glucose transport*

Controversy exists as to whether basal glucose transport in adipocytes can be changed by exercise training. Some studies show an increase in basal glucose transport per adipocyte in trained compared with sedentary age-matched female rats having similar adipocyte sizes.[60] In contrast, others show a decrease in basal glucose transport per adipocyte in trained compared with sedentary age-matched female rats, but an increase in glucose transport compared with sedentary younger control rats.[56] Hirshman et al.[56] normalized glucose transport data and expressed them per adipocyte surface area to be able to compare adipocytes of different size. Expressed in this way, trained rats did not differ from age-matched control rats. Vinten and Galbo[50] expressed glucose transport per adipocyte and found no difference in basal glucose transport between trained and sedentary age-matched male rats (of which some were food-restricted to have comparable adipocyte size with trained rats). In male rats, a difference in basal glucose transport expressed per adipocyte between trained and sedentary age-matched or younger control rats was not found (see Figure 4.2).[58] Basal glucose transport expressed per adipocyte surface area was higher in trained compared with sedentary age-matched rats (see Figure 4.2).[58] In all the previously mentioned studies, glucose transport was measured 40 to 44 hr after the last exercise bout and, accordingly, the acute effect of exercise probably did not affect the results.

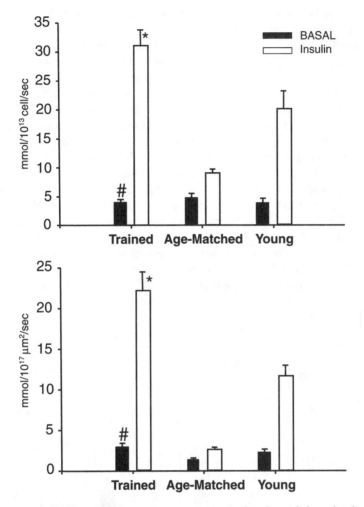

*Figure 4.2*   3-O-[14C]methylglucose transport in isolated epididymal adipocytes from swim-trained rats (*n* = 10) or rats serving as sedentary control groups matched with respect to age (~14 wk old, *n* = 9) or adipocyte volume (~6 wk old, *n* = 8). Values are means ± SE. The symbol * indicates *p* < 0.05 vs. sedentary control groups; # indicates *p* < 0.05 vs. age-matched control group. (Data from Stallknecht, B. et al., *Am. J. Physiol.*, 265, E128, 1993.)

The only human study comparing glucose transport in trained vs. sedentary subjects was performed by Rodnick et al.,[77] who measured basal glucose transport in subcutaneous, abdominal adipocytes from male runners and sedentary control subjects. Basal glucose transport expressed per adipocyte did not differ between trained and sedentary subjects, but because the adipocytes were significantly smaller in the trained subjects, basal glucose transport per adipocyte surface area was probably increased in the trained subjects.[77]

Craig and co-workers[19,55,61,63,64,67] measured glucose uptake in adipocytes by the glucose analog 2-deoxyglucose. Because this glucose analog is phosphorylated in the adipocyte (but not further metabolized), it measures not only glucose transport but also glucose phosphorylation.[82] Accordingly, 2-deoxyglucose uptake is not a reliable measure of glucose transport.[82] In most studies, Craig and co-workers[19,55,61,63,67] examined parametrial adipocytes from trained and sedentary female rats, but in one study they examined epididymal adipocytes from male rats.[64] Adipocytes were studied 24 hr after the last bout of exercise (in trained rats), and in all studies but one,[55] basal glucose uptake per adipocyte was increased in trained animals.[19,61,63,64,67] Studies included examination of trained and sedentary pregnant[63] and old[64] rats. Craig and co-workers[61,67] also examined the effect of detraining on glucose uptake, and it is notable that basal glucose uptake remained elevated in 7-day detrained rats compared with sedentary control rats, as these groups of rats did not differ in adipocyte size (see Figure 4.3).[67]

In conclusion, due to contradictory results, it is not clear if basal glucose transport is increased, decreased, or unchanged in adipocytes from trained compared with sedentary age-matched individuals. Most studies, however, found an increased basal glucose uptake expressed per adipocyte in trained compared with sedentary rats.

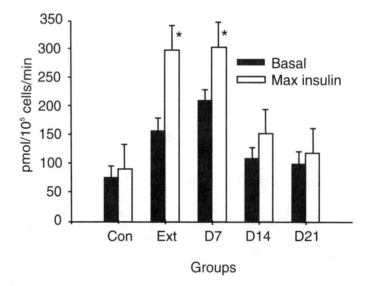

*Figure 4.3*    2-[³H]deoxyglucose uptake in isolated parametrial adipocytes from sedentary control, trained, and 7-, 14- and 21-day detrained rats (each group contained 8 to 12 animals). Basal and maximal insulin represent glucose uptake with no and 1000 $\mu$U/mL insulin, respectively, present in the incubation medium; the symbol * indicates $p < 0.05$ vs. corresponding basal group. (Reprinted from *Mech. Ageing Dev.*, 57, 49, Craig, B.W. et al., Copyright 1991, with permission from Elsevier Science.)

### 4.5.1.2 Effect of insulin

Insulin-stimulated glucose transport per adipocyte is, without exception, higher in trained compared with sedentary age-matched rats (Figure 4.2)[50,56,58] and humans.[77] The fold increase in glucose transport induced by a maximal insulin concentration (estimated from graphs) was much higher in adipocytes from trained rats (seven- to tenfold) compared with adipocytes from sedentary age-matched rats (one- to eightfold) (Figure 4.2).[50,56,58,60] In the human study, the fold increase in glucose transport during insulin-stimulation was significantly higher in adipocytes from trained compared with sedentary men (approximately three- and twofold, respectively).[77] Moreover, the insulin-stimulated glucose transport per adipocyte was higher in trained rats compared with younger (Figure 4.2)[56,58] and food-restricted control rats.[50] Also, when expressed per adipocyte surface area, the insulin-stimulated glucose transport was higher in trained compared with both sedentary age-matched and younger control rats (Figure 4.2).[56,58] As little as 4 days of swimming was sufficient to increase the insulin-stimulated glucose transport in epididymal adipocytes from male rats when measured 18 to 22 hr after the last exercise bout.[71]

In addition, maximally insulin-stimulated 2-deoxyglucose uptake per adipocyte is consistently elevated in trained compared with sedentary age-matched rats with estimated insulin-stimulated fold increases of 1 to 5 and 0.1 to 0.5, respectively (Figure 4.3).[55,61,64,67] In many studies, the 2-deoxyglucose uptake was measured at a number of insulin concentrations both in the physiological and in the supraphysiological insulin concentration range, and glucose uptake was higher in adipocytes from trained compared with sedentary rats also at physiological insulin concentrations.[19,55,61,63,64] The insulin-stimulated 2-deoxyglucose uptake in adipocytes decreased with detraining, but the training effect was relatively persistent as glucose uptake was still higher compared with sedentary rats 7 days (Figure 4.3)[67] and 9 days[61] after the last exercise bout.

The authors studied the mechanism behind the training-induced increase in insulin-stimulated glucose transport in adipocytes[70] by swim-training rats that were either adrenodemedullated or sham-adrenodemedullated, and either underwent unilateral abdominal sympathectomy or were sham-sympathectomized. Training increased insulin-stimulated glucose transport in epididymal adipocytes, and neither adrenodemedullation nor sympathetic denervation affected the increase, indicating that adrenergic activity is not important for the training-induced increase in insulin-stimulated glucose transport in adipocytes.[70] Interestingly, the decrease in adipocyte size with training was also not influenced by adrenodemedullation or sympathetic denervation.[70]

In conclusion, insulin-stimulated glucose transport is increased in adipocytes from trained compared with sedentary rats and humans.

## 4.5.2   Number of insulin receptors

Insulin must bind to its receptor on the plasma membrane before glucose transport is stimulated, so it is interesting to know if exercise training increases the number of insulin receptors in adipocytes. Unfortunately, insulin binding per adipocyte can be both increased[19,50] and unchanged[60] in trained compared with sedentary, age-matched rats. Also, Wirth et al.[68] found no change in insulin binding in trained compared with sedentary, age-matched, freely eating or food-restricted rats, but they did not state how insulin binding was expressed. However, Craig et al.[19] calculated that the increased insulin binding found in their study was due to an increased number of insulin receptors. In another study, obese type II diabetic and non-diabetic human male and female subjects were trained for 3 months, and fat biopsies were obtained from the abdominal, subcutaneous adipose tissue before and after training.[76] Insulin binding per adipocyte was unchanged by training in both diabetic and non-diabetic subjects.[76]

## 4.5.3   Number of glucose transporters

The increased insulin-stimulated glucose transport in adipocytes from trained compared with sedentary individuals could be due to an increased number of glucose transporters in the adipocyte plasma membrane of trained individuals and/or an increase in the activity of glucose transporters. In the non-stimulated state, most of the glucose transporters are stored in the interior of the adipocyte (in low-density microsomes) and, upon stimulation by insulin, a fraction of these glucose transporters are recruited to the plasma membrane.[83,84] The number of glucose transporters in the plasma membrane and in the low-density microsome fractions of homogenized adipocytes can be estimated by cytochalasin B binding.[84,85] In the non-stimulated state, the number of glucose transporters (measured by cytochalasin B binding) per adipocyte in the low-density microsome fraction was higher in trained compared with sedentary, age-matched, food-restricted[62] and freely eating rats.[56] In the insulin-stimulated state, the number of glucose transporters per adipocyte in the plasma membrane was higher in trained compared with sedentary, age-matched, food-restricted,[62] and younger control rats,[56] but not compared with sedentary, age-matched, freely eating rats.[56] Adipocytes from trained rats were significantly smaller than adipocytes from sedentary, age-matched rats, and when expressed per adipocyte surface area, a greater number of glucose transporters were observed in the plasma membrane in the insulin-stimulated state in trained compared with sedentary, age-matched rats.[56]

In the late 1980s, it became clear that many classes of glucose transporters exist, of which two (termed GLUT-4 and GLUT-1) are present in adipocytes.[20,21,86,87] GLUT-4 is responsible for most of the insulin-stimulated glucose transport in adipocytes, and it is much more abundant than GLUT-1 in adipocytes.[20,21,86] The authors, and others, found that the total number of

GLUT-4 was increased in epididymal adipocytes from trained compared with sedentary, younger control rats when expressed per cell (see Figure 4.4).[57,58] Furthermore, we found that, when normalized for adipocyte size, the total number of GLUT-4 was greater in trained compared with both sedentary, age-matched and younger control rats (Figure 4.4).[58] In contrast, training did not increase the number of GLUT-1 per cell[57,58] or per adipocyte surface area.[58]

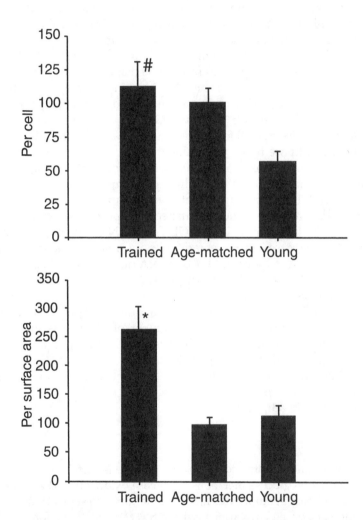

*Figure 4.4*    Quantitation of GLUT-4 protein in isolated epididymal adipocytes from swim-trained rats ($n = 11$) or rats serving as sedentary control groups matched with respect to age (~14 wk old, $n = 10$) or adipocyte volume (~6 wk old, $n = 10$). GLUT-4 protein was determined by western blot, and values are expressed as percent of mean value in sedentary, age-matched control group. Values are means ± SE. The symbol * indicates $p < 0.05$ vs. sedentary control groups; # indicates $p < 0.05$ vs. younger control group. (Data from Stallknecht, B. et al., *Am. J. Physiol.*, 265, E128, 1993.)

Hirshman et al.[57] measured GLUT-4 and GLUT-1 in plasma membranes and low-density microsomes separately. In plasma membranes, they found an increase in basal and insulin-stimulated GLUT-4 protein expressed per adipocyte as well as per adipocyte surface area in trained compared with sedentary, younger control rats.[57] Compared with sedentary, age-matched rats, GLUT-4 per adipocyte surface area was greater in trained rats.[57] In low-density microsomes, basal GLUT-4 per adipocyte and per surface area are elevated in trained compared with sedentary, age-matched rats, but not compared with sedentary younger control rats.[57] Training did not change GLUT-1 in plasma membranes or in low-density microsomes.[57]

The authors measured the amount of mRNA coding for GLUT-4 and GLUT-1 in epididymal adipocytes from trained and sedentary male rats and found a large increase in GLUT-4 mRNA in trained compared with sedentary, age-matched rats, both when expressed per adipocyte and per adipocyte surface area (see Figure 4.5);[58] however, GLUT-1 mRNA was not increased by training.[58] In mice trained for 3 weeks, an increase in both GLUT-4 protein and mRNA in adipose tissue was found.[88]

During insulin stimulation, 4-day-swim-trained rats had an increased number of cell surface GLUT-4 per adipocyte compared with sedentary rats, whereas GLUT-1 did not differ between groups.[71] Seven-day-running-trained rats had mesenteric and subcutaneous adipose tissue removed immediately after the last exercise bout.[69] GLUT-4 mRNA expressed per amount of total RNA decreased in mesenteric adipose tissue of trained compared with sedentary rats, whereas GLUT-4 mRNA did not change by training in subcutaneous adipose tissue.[69] Most likely, the last acute bout of exercise influenced the results of the latter study.

In conclusion, training increases the total number of glucose transporters in adipocytes. In the basal state, the number of GLUT-4 is increased by training in the membrane depot in the interior of the adipocyte, whereas in the insulin-stimulated state, training increases the number of GLUT-4 in the adipocyte plasma membrane. Training does not increase the number of GLUT-1. Likewise, exercise training increases GLUT-4 mRNA, but not GLUT-1 mRNA, in adipocytes.

### 4.5.4   In vitro *glucose metabolism*

After entry of glucose into the adipocyte, glucose is metabolized. The effect of training on total glucose metabolism, glucose oxidation, and glucose incorporation into lipids in adipocytes has been examined in several studies. Studies included rats trained by various swimming[19,46,50,55,61,62,67] and forced[44,54,59,60,63] and voluntary[56,64-66] treadmill protocols. Furthermore, some studies examined epididymal adipocytes from male rats,[44,46,50,54,59,62,64,65] and other studies examined parametrial adipocytes from female rats,[19,55,56,60,61,63,66,67] but no studies compared responses in males and females directly. No apparent differences between sexes in training responses were observed.

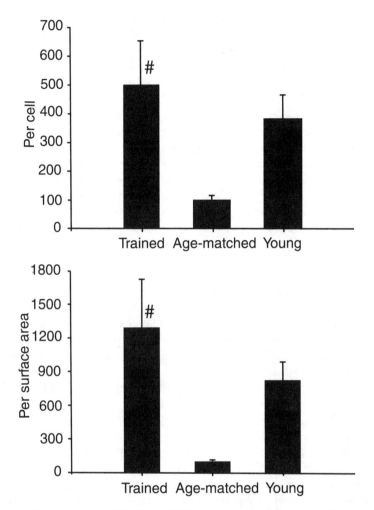

***Figure 4.5*** Quantitation of GLUT-4 mRNA in isolated epididymal adipocytes from swim-trained rats ($n = 10$) or rats serving as sedentary control groups matched with respect to age (~14 weeks old, $n = 10$) or adipocyte volume (~6 wk old, $n = 5$). GLUT-4 mRNA was determined by slot blot, and values are expressed as percent of mean value in sedentary age-matched control group. Values are means ± SE. The symbol # indicates $p < 0.05$ vs. age-matched control group. (Data from Stallknecht, B. et al., *Am. J. Physiol.*, 265, E128, 1993.)

### 4.5.4.1 *Basal glucose metabolism*

In the non-stimulated state, total glucose utilization will increase[60] and decrease[54,56] in trained compared with sedentary age-matched rats when expressed per adipocyte. Glucose utilization per adipocyte was higher when trained rats were compared with sedentary younger control rats.[56] When expressed per adipocyte surface area, basal glucose utilization was increased[66] or unchanged[56] in trained compared with sedentary, age-matched rats. Training did not change basal glucose utilization per adipocyte in obese rats,[60] but basal glucose utilization per adipocyte surface area was increased by training in rats with impaired glucose tolerance.[66]

The influence of training on basal glucose oxidation in rat adipocytes also varied in different studies. When expressed per adipocyte, most found an increase,[55,60,61,64] some found no change,[19,59,63] and some found a decrease[65] in trained compared with sedentary, age-matched rats. Craig and Foley[55] measured glucose oxidation both via the pentose phosphate pathway and via glycolysis and found a training-induced increase in glucose oxidation per adipocyte in both pathways. Four and 9 days of detraining did not reduce basal glucose oxidation to sedentary levels.[61] When glucose oxidation is expressed per adipocyte surface area, some studies show an increase[66] and others show no change[59] with training in rats. Training also increased basal glucose oxidation in obese rats when expressed per adipocyte[60] and in rats with impaired glucose tolerance when expressed per adipocyte surface area.[66]

Incorporation of glucose into total TG (i.e., into both the fatty acid and the glycerol part of TG) was decreased[46,65] or not changed[50,59,62] per adipocyte in trained compared with sedentary, age-matched rats. However, training increased glucose incorporation into TG when expressed per adipocyte surface area.[59] Training of both lean and obese rats increased glucose incorporation into the fatty acid part of TG when expressed per adipocyte.[60] Likewise, in normal rats and in rats with impaired glucose tolerance, training increased glucose incorporation into the fatty acid part of TG and did not change glucose incorporation into the glycerol part of TG when expressed per adipocyte surface area.[66]

In trained compared with sedentary, lean men, some researchers have found an increase in basal glucose conversion to TG per adipocyte,[73] whereas others have found no difference.[72,74] The study by Savard et al.,[73] in which an increase was found in trained subjects, examined male marathon runners (i.e., very well-trained subjects), and the increase was still present after matching trained and sedentary men for adipocyte size.[73] In another study, Savard et al.[75] trained males and females for 20 weeks and found an increased basal glucose conversion to TG per adipocyte in male, but not in female, subjects. Krotkiewski et al.[76] studied obese, type II diabetic and non-diabetic subjects before and after 3 months of training and found no change in basal glucose conversion to TG per adipocyte in either group.

In conclusion, many studies have examined the effect of training on basal *in vitro* glucose metabolism in adipocytes, especially in rats, but results are not consistent. This indicates that exercise training most likely has no major influence on basal glucose metabolism in adipocytes.

### 4.5.4.2   Effect of insulin and epinephrine

Exercise training increased insulin-stimulated total glucose utilization per adipocyte in some[56,60] but not all studies.[54] When compared to sedentary, younger control rats,[56] and when expressed per adipocyte surface area, insulin-stimulated glucose utilization is consistently increased.[56,66] Moreover, training increases insulin-stimulated glucose utilization per adipocyte in obese rats[60] and in rats with impaired glucose tolerance.[66] Insulin sensitivity (indicated by the concentration of insulin resulting in half-maximal stimulation of glucose utilization) is not changed by training in adipocytes of lean,[60,66] obese,[60] or glucose intolerant rats.[66]

Insulin-stimulated glucose oxidation per adipocyte was higher in trained compared with sedentary, age-matched rats in most studies.[19,55,60,61,63,64,67] Nevertheless, some found no change in insulin-stimulated glucose oxidation per adipocyte after training.[59,65] However, although Lawrence et al.[65] found no increase in insulin-stimulated glucose oxidation after training in absolute terms, during insulin-stimulation they found a percentage increase compared with basal in trained rats. Training increased the insulin-stimulated glucose oxidation both via the pentose phosphate pathway and via glycolysis.[55,67] Detraining for 4, 7, and 9 days did not reduce insulin-stimulated glucose oxidation to sedentary levels, but after 14 days of detraining, glucose oxidation was no longer increased.[61,67] When insulin-stimulated glucose oxidation is expressed per adipocyte surface area, some researchers have found an increase[66] and some have found no change[59] in trained compared with sedentary, age-matched rats. In addition, training increased insulin-stimulated glucose oxidation in obese rats[60] and in rats with impaired glucose tolerance.[66] Training either increased[50,62] or did not change[44,46,59,65] insulin-stimulated incorporation of glucose into total TG. However, when expressed per adipocyte surface area[59] or when expressed as a percentage increase during insulin stimulation,[46,65] adipocytes from trained rats had a higher insulin-stimulated glucose incorporation into TG compared with adipocytes from sedentary, age-matched rats. Training increased the insulin-stimulated glucose incorporation into the fatty acid part of TG and did not change the insulin-stimulated glucose incorporation into the glycerol part of TG in adipocytes from lean,[60,66] obese,[60] and glucose intolerant rats.[66]

In human studies, an increase in insulin-stimulated glucose conversion to TG per adipocyte,[73] or no difference,[72,74] was found in trained compared with sedentary subjects. In the study by Savard et al.,[73] the increase was still present after matching trained and sedentary men for adipocyte size. Savard et al.[75] found a gender difference in the training response for insulin-stimulated glucose conversion to TG, with an increase after training in males and no change in females (see Figure 4.6). In addition, training increased the insulin-stimulated glucose conversion to TG per adipocyte in obese, type II diabetic subjects, but not in obese non-diabetic subjects.[76]

In conclusion, most studies show that exercise training increases the insulin-stimulated total glucose utilization in adipocytes. Training, however, does not change insulin sensitivity with respect to glucose utilization in adipocytes. The fraction of glucose that is oxidized may also increase training in insulin-stimulated adipocytes. It is less clear if training increases insulin-stimulated glucose incorporation into total TG, but glucose incorporation into the fatty acid part of TG may increase.

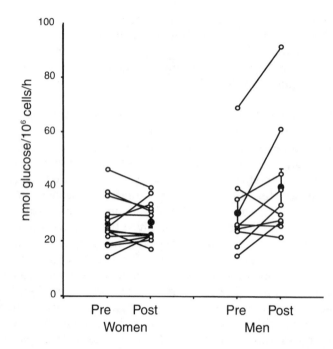

**Figure 4.6**   Maximal insulin-stimulated glucose conversion to triacylglycerol pre- and post-training in women ($n = 13$) and men ($n = 10$). Individual values and means ± SE are presented. (From Savard, R. et al., *J. Appl. Physiol.*, 58, 230, 1985. With permission.)

Only one study examined the effect of training on epinephrine-stimulated glucose utilization in rat adipocytes, and in that study a training-induced decrease was found.[54]

### 4.5.5   *In vivo glucose metabolism*

#### 4.5.5.1   *Basal glucose metabolism*

In the overnight fasted state, adipose tissue takes up glucose[28,79,81,89] and releases lactate[28,29,81,90] *in vivo*. Glucose uptake is low because the arterio-venous glucose difference over abdominal, subcutaneous adipose tissue is small (~0.1 m$M$),[89] and the adipose tissue blood flow is low (~3 mL 100 g$^{-1}$ min$^{-1}$).[28,81] The fact that adipose tissue is of minor importance in whole-body glucose metabolism is also suggested by Björntorp et al.,[18] who demonstrated that adipose tissue took up only 0.5 and 2% of an intravenous glucose load in lean and obese subjects, respectively.

James et al.[78] trained male rats by forced running for 7 weeks and found no significant effect of training on basal glucose uptake per gram of epididymal adipose tissue measured by the glucose analog 2-deoxyglucose. This study also measured *in vivo* glucose incorporation into the fatty acid and glycerol parts of TG, respectively, in adipose tissue. The study found lower glucose incorporation into the fatty acid part with no change in glucose incorporation into the glycerol part in trained compared with sedentary rats.[78] The authors studied athletes and sedentary male subjects using microdialysis and also found no difference in basal glucose uptake per gram of subcutaneous, abdominal adipose tissue between groups.[28]

A study by Yang et al.[80] indicated no difference in lactate production in inguinal adipose tissue between trained and sedentary rats because no difference was found in microdialysate lactate concentrations between groups. Because neither arterial lactate concentrations nor adipose tissue blood flow were studied, conclusions are difficult to draw. The authors also estimated lactate release from adipose tissue using microdialysis and found no difference in basal lactate output per gram of adipose tissue in athletes compared with sedentary male subjects.[28] In conclusion, training does not change basal adipose tissue glucose uptake or lactate release *in vivo*.

### 4.5.5.2   *Effect of insulin and epinephrine*

The arteriovenous glucose difference across human abdominal, subcutaneous adipose tissue was found to increase slightly during a hyperinsulinemic, euglycemic clamp.[29] The authors found no change in adipose tissue blood flow during a hyperinsulinemic, euglycemic clamp.[81] Thus, the insulin-stimulated increase in glucose uptake in adipose tissue must be small. Modest insulin stimulation of adipose tissue glucose uptake is indirectly suggested by DeFronzo et al.,[91] who estimated that skeletal muscle accounts for 85% of the total insulin-stimulated glucose uptake in humans.

Training increases insulin-stimulated, whole-body glucose uptake in humans,[92,93] and both sensitivity and responsiveness of insulin-stimulated glucose uptake are increased in human muscle by training.[94] Using microdialysis, the authors found an insulin-stimulated increase in glucose uptake in abdominal, subcutaneous adipose tissue in male athletes, but no significant stimulation of glucose uptake by insulin in sedentary males.[81] In addition, the authors studied insulin-stimulated glucose uptake in retroperitoneal, parametrial, mesenteric, and subcutaneous adipose tissues in trained and sedentary, age-matched rats by both microdialysis and *in vivo* 2-deoxyglucose (see Figure 4.7).[79] The authors found, with both techniques, a higher insulin-stimulated glucose uptake per gram of adipose tissue in trained compared with sedentary rats in all tissues, with no significant difference between adipose tissues studied (Figure 4.7).[79] Previously, James et al.[78] also found an increased *in vivo* insulin-stimulated glucose uptake per gram of epididymal adipose tissue in trained compared with sedentary, age-matched rats. Moreover, they found a significantly higher glucose conversion to free fatty acid (FFA) in the adipose tissue of the trained rats.[78]

Neither the authors[81] nor Yang et al.[80] found a difference between trained and sedentary individuals in adipose tissue microdialysate lactate concentration during insulin stimulation, indicating no difference in insulin-stimulated lactate production in adipose tissue between groups. Thus, training increases insulin-stimulated glucose uptake in adipose tissue *in vivo* but does not change insulin-stimulated lactate release.

Epinephrine stimulates *in vivo* glucose uptake in and lactate release from adipose tissue.[28] However, we found no difference between male athletes and sedentary males in epinephrine-stimulated glucose uptake in subcutaneous,

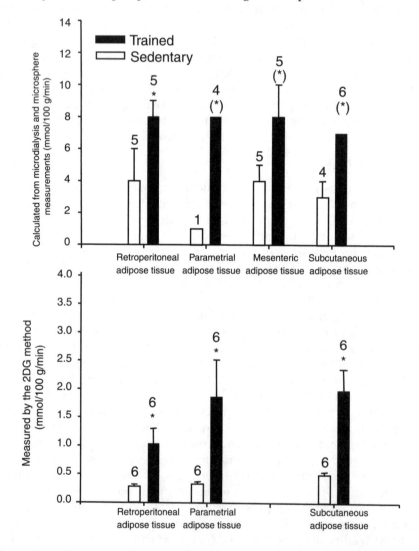

*Figure 4.7*  Glucose uptake rate calculated from microdialysis and microsphere measurements (top) or measured by 2-[³H]deoxyglucose (2-DG) method (bottom) in various adipose tissues in trained and sedentary rats at 60–90 min (top) or at 90–120 min (bottom) of a 120-min hyperinsulinemic (1.67 mU insulin kg⁻¹ min⁻¹), euglycemic clamp. Values are means ± SE. The symbol * indicates $p < 0.05$ vs. sedentary rats; (*) indicates $p < 0.1$ vs. sedentary rats. Number of observations is shown. (Modified from Enevoldsen, L.H. et al., *Am. J. Physiol. Endocrinol. Metab.*, 278, E25, 2000. With permission.)

abdominal adipose tissue estimated by microdialysis technique.[28] Moreover, in the same study the authors found no difference between trained and sedentary subjects in lactate output from adipose tissue. Thus, training does not change epinephrine-stimulated glucose uptake in and lactate release from adipose tissue *in vivo*.

## 4.6   Conclusions

1. An acute bout of exercise appears to decrease basal and insulin-stimulated glucose transport and *de novo* lipogenesis in adipose tissue of normal-weight individuals, but few studies have examined the effect of acute exercise on glucose metabolism in adipose tissue.
2. It is not clear if basal glucose transport is increased, decreased, or unchanged in adipocytes from trained compared with sedentary age-matched individuals because contradicting results have been found. Most studies, however, have found an increased basal glucose uptake in adipocytes from trained compared with sedentary rats. Insulin-stimulated glucose transport is increased in adipocytes from trained compared with sedentary rats and humans, which cannot be ascribed to the sympathetic nervous system.
3. It is not clear if exercise training increases or does not change the number of insulin receptors in adipocytes.
4. Training increases the total number of glucose transporters in adipocytes. In the basal state, the number of GLUT-4 is increased by training in the membrane depot in the interior of the adipocyte, whereas in the insulin-stimulated state training increases the number of GLUT-4 in the adipocyte plasma membrane. Exercise training also increases GLUT-4 mRNA in adipose tissue. Training does not affect the number or mRNA of GLUT-1.
5. Although many studies have examined the effect of exercise training on basal *in vitro* glucose metabolism in adipocytes, especially in rats, the results are not clear. Most studies have shown that training increases the insulin-stimulated total glucose utilization in adipocytes. Training, however, does not change insulin sensitivity with respect to glucose utilization in adipocytes. The fraction of glucose that is oxidized also seems to be increased by training in insulin-stimulated adipocytes. It is less clear if training increases insulin-stimulated glucose incorporation into total TG, but glucose incorporation into the fatty acid part of TG may increase.
6. Exercise training does not change basal adipose tissue *in vivo* glucose uptake or lactate release. Training increases insulin-stimulated glucose uptake in adipose tissue *in vivo*, but does not change insulin-stimulated lactate release. Training does not change epinephrine-stimulated glucose uptake and lactate release from adipose tissue *in vivo*.

## Acknowledgments

The author is supported by the Danish National Research Foundation (504-14).

## References

1. Ivy, J.L., Role of carbohydrate in physical activity, *Clin. Sports Med.*, 18, 469, 1999.
2. Hargreaves, M., 1997 Sir William Refshauge Lecture. Skeletal muscle glucose metabolism during exercise: implications for health and performance, *J. Sci. Med. Sport*, 1, 195, 1998.
3. Holloszy, J.O., Kohrt, W.M., and Hansen, P.A., The regulation of carbohydrate and fat metabolism during and after exercise, *Front. Biosci.*, 3, D1011, 1998.
4. De Glisezinski, I. et al., Endurance training changes in lipolytic responsiveness of obese adipose tissue, *Am. J. Physiol. Endocrinol. Metab.*, 275, E951, 1998.
5. Shepherd, R.E. and Bah, M.D., Cyclic AMP regulation of fuel metabolism during exercise: regulation of adipose tissue lipolysis during exercise, *Med. Sci. Sports Exerc.*, 20, 531, 1988.
6. Turcotte, L.P., Role of fats in exercise: types and quality, *Clin. Sports Med.*, 18, 485, 1999.
7. Horowitz, J.F. and Klein, S., Lipid metabolism during endurance exercise, *Am. J. Clin. Nutr.*, 72, 558S, 2000.
8. Frayn, K.N., Regulation of fatty acid delivery in vivo, *Adv. Exp. Med. Biol.*, 441, 171, 1998.
9. Lehninger, A.L., *Principles of Biochemistry*, Worth Publishers, New York, 1982.
10. Frayn, K.N., *Metabolic Regulation: A Human Perspective*, Portland Press, London, 1996.
11. Potts, J.L. et al., Peripheral triacylglycerol extraction in the fasting and postprandial states, *Clin. Sci.*, 81, 621, 1991.
12. Frayn, K.N., Studies of human adipose tissue in vivo, in *Energy Metabolism: Tissue Determinants and Cellular Corollaries*, J.M. Kinney and H.N. Tucker, Eds., Raven Press, New York, 1992.
13. Acheson, K.J., Flatt, J.P., and Jequier, E., Glycogen synthesis versus lipogenesis after a 500-gram carbohydrate meal in man, *Metabolism*, 31, 1234, 1982.
14. Pozza, G., Ghidoni, A., and Basilico, C., Glucose uptake and gas exchange in human adipose tisssue incubated in vitro, *Lancet*, 1, 836, 1963.
15. Robinson, J. and Newsholme, E.A., Glycerol kinase activities in rat heart and adipose tissue, *Biochem. J.*, 104, 2C, 1967.
16. Koschinsky, T. and Gries, F.A., Glycerol kinase and lipolysis in human adipose tissue in relation to relative body weight, *Hoppe-Seylers Zeitschrift fur Physiologische Chemie*, 352, 430, 1971.
17. Frayn, K.N., Humphreys, S.M., and Coppack, S.W., Fuel selection in white adipose tissue, *Proc. Nutr. Soc.*, 54, 177, 1995.
18. Björntorp, P. et al., The glucose uptake of human adipose tissue in obesity, *Eur. J. Clin. Invest.*, 1, 480, 1971.
19. Craig, B.W. et al., Adaptation of fat cells to exercise: response of glucose uptake and oxidation to insulin, *J. Appl. Physiol.*, 51, 1500, 1981.
20. Mueckler, M., Facilitative glucose transporters, *Eur. J. Biochem.*, 219, 713, 1994.

21. Kahn, B.B., Lilly lecture 1995. Glucose transport: pivotal step in insulin action, *Diabetes*, 45, 1644, 1996.
22. Rigden, D.J. et al., Human adipose tissue glycogen levels and responses to carbohydrate feeding, *Eur. J. Clin. Nutr.*, 44, 689, 1990.
23. Coppack, S.W., Jensen, M.D., and Miles, J.M., In vivo regulation of lipolysis in humans, *J. Lipid Res.*, 35, 177, 1994.
24. Vinten, J., Gliemann, J., and Osterlind, K., Exchange of 3-O-methylglucose in isolated fat cells. Concentration dependence and effect of insulin, *J. Biol. Chem.*, 251, 794, 1976.
25. Rasmussen, M.J. and Clausen, T., The stimulating effect of 3′,5′-(cyclic)adenosine monophosphate and lipolytic hormones on 3-O-methylglucose transport and $^{45}Ca^{2+}$ release in adipocytes and skeletal muscle of the rat, *Biochim. Biophys. Acta*, 693, 389, 1982.
26. Ludvigsen, C., Jarett, L., and McDonald, J.M., The characterization of catecholamine stimulation of glucose transport by rat adipocytes and isolated plasma membranes, *Endocrinology*, 106, 786, 1980.
27. Arner, P. et al., Effects of lipolytic and antilipolytic agents on glucose transport in human fat cells, *Int. J. Obesity*, 15, 327, 1991.
28. Stallknecht, B. et al., Effect of training on epinephrine-stimulated lipolysis determined by microdialysis in human adipose tissue, *Am. J. Physiol.*, 269, E1059, 1995.
29. Coppack, S.W. et al., Effects of insulin on human adipose tissue metabolism in vivo, *Clin. Sci.*, 77, 663, 1989.
30. James, D.E., Burleigh, K.M., and Kraegen, E.W., Time dependence of insulin action in muscle and adipose tissue in the rat in vivo. An increasing response in adipose tissue with time, *Diabetes*, 34, 1049, 1985.
31. Galbo, H., *Hormonal and Metabolic Adaptation to Exercise*, Thieme-Stratton, New York, 1983.
32. Frayn, K.N. et al., Metabolic characteristics of human adipose tissue in vivo, *Clin. Sci.*, 76, 509, 1989.
33. Frayn, K.N., Coppack, S.W., and Humphreys, S.M., Subcutaneous adipose tissue metabolism studied by local catheterization, *Int. J. Obesity*, 17, S18, 1993.
34. Lönnroth, P., Jansson, P.A., and Smith, U., A microdialysis method allowing characterization of intercellular water space in humans, *Am. J. Physiol.*, 253, E228, 1987.
35. Arner, P. et al., Microdialysis of adipose tissue and blood for in vivo lipolysis studies, *Am. J. Physiol.*, 255, E737, 1988.
36. Arner, P., Microdialysis: use in human exercise studies, *Proc. Nutr. Soc.*, 58, 913, 1999.
37. Lönnroth, P., Microdialysis in adipose tissue and skeletal muscle, *Horm. Metab. Res.*, 29, 344, 1997.
38. Lafontan, M. and Arner, P., Application of in situ microdialysis to measure metabolic and vascular responses in adipose tissue, *Trends Pharmacol. Sci.*, 17, 309, 1996.
39. Arner, P., Techniques for the measurement of white adipose tissue metabolism: a practical guide, *Int. J. Obesity*, 19, 435, 1995.
40. Arner, P. and Bülow, J., Assessment of adipose tissue metabolism in man: comparison of Fick and microdialysis techniques, *Clin. Sci.*, 85, 247, 1993.

41. Mulla, N.A., Simonsen, L., and Bülow, J., Post-exercise adipose tissue and skeletal muscle lipid metabolism in humans: the effects of exercise intensity, *J. Physiol. Lond.*, 524(part 3), 919, 2000.

42. Koivisto, V.A. and Yki-Järvinen, H., Effect of exercise on insulin binding and glucose transport in adipocytes of normal humans, *J. Appl. Physiol.*, 63, 1319, 1987.

43. Savard, R. et al., Acute effects of endurance exercise on human adipose tissue metabolism, *Metabolism*, 36, 480, 1987.

44. Askew, E.W. et al., Response of lipogenesis and fatty acid synthetase to physical training and exhaustive exercise in rats, *Lipids*, 10, 491, 1975.

45. Askew, E.W. et al., Lipogenesis and glyceride synthesis in the rat: response to diet and exercise, *J. Nutr.*, 105, 190, 1975.

46. Kral, J.G. et al., The effects of physical exercise on fat cell metabolism in the rat, *Acta Physiol. Scand.*, 90, 664, 1974.

47. Nagasawa, J., Sato, Y., and Ishiko, T., Time course of in vivo insulin sensitivity after a single bout of exercise in rats, *Int. J. Sports Med.*, 12, 399, 1991.

48. Burstein, R. et al., Glucose uptake by adipocytes of obese rats: effect of one bout of acute exercise, *Can. J. Physiol. Pharmacol.*, 70, 1473, 1992.

49. Oscai, L.B., The role of exercise in weight control, *Exerc. Sport Sci. Rev.*, 1, 103, 1973.

50. Vinten, J. and Galbo, H., Effect of physical training on transport and metabolism of glucose in adipocytes, *Am. J. Physiol.*, 244, E129, 1983.

51. Björntorp, P. and Sjöström, L., The composition and metabolism in vitro of adipose tissue fat cells of different sizes, *Eur. J. Clin. Invest.*, 2, 78, 1972.

52. Holm, G. et al., Effects of age and cell size on rat adipose tissue metabolism, *J. Lipid Res.*, 16, 461, 1975.

53. Gommers, A. and Dehez-Delhaye, M., Effect of maturation and senescence on carbohydrate utilization and insulin responsiveness of rat adipose tissue, *Acta Diabetol. Lat.*, 16, 317, 1979.

54. Owens, J.L. et al., Influence of moderate exercise on adipocyte metabolism and hormonal responsiveness, *J. Appl. Physiol.*, 43, 425, 1977.

55. Craig, B.W. and Foley, P.J., Effects of cell size and exercise on glucose uptake and metabolism in adipocytes of female rats, *J. Appl. Physiol.*, 57, 1120, 1984.

56. Hirshman, M.F. et al., Exercise training increases the number of glucose transporters in rat adipose cells, *Am. J. Physiol.*, 257, E520, 1989.

57. Hirshman, M.F. et al., Exercise training increases GLUT-4 protein in rat adipose cells, *Am. J. Physiol.*, 264, E882, 1993.

58. Stallknecht, B. et al., Effect of physical training on glucose transporter protein and mRNA levels in rat adipocytes, *Am. J. Physiol.*, 265, E128, 1993.

59. Palmer, W.K. and Tipton, C.M., Effect of training on adipocyte glucose metabolism and insulin responsiveness, *Fed. Proc.*, 33, 1964, 1974.

60. Wardzala, L.J. et al., Physical training of lean and genetically obese Zucker rats: effect on fat cell metabolism, *Am. J. Physiol.*, 243, E418, 1982.

61. Craig, B.W., Thompson, K., and Holloszy, J.O., Effects of stopping training on size and response to insulin of fat cells in female rats, *J. Appl. Physiol.*, 54, 571, 1983.

62. Vinten, J. et al., Effect of physical training on glucose transporters in fat cell fractions, *Biochim. Biophys. Acta*, 841, 223, 1985.

63. Craig, B.W. and Treadway, J., Glucose uptake and oxidation in fat cells of trained and sedentary pregnant rats, *J. Appl. Physiol.*, 60, 1704, 1986.

64. Craig, B.W., Garthwaite, S.M., and Holloszy, J.O., Adipocyte insulin resistance: effects of aging, obesity, exercise, and food restriction, *J. Appl. Physiol.*, 62, 95, 1987.

65. Lawrence, Jr., J.C. et al., Effects of aging and exercise on insulin action in rat adipocytes are correlated with changes in fat cell volume, *J. Gerontol.*, 44, B88, 1989.

66. Goodyear, L.J. et al., Exercise training normalizes glucose metabolism in a rat model of impaired glucose tolerance, *Metabolism*, 40, 455, 1991.

67. Craig, B.W. et al., The influence of training-detraining upon the heart, muscle and adipose tissue of female rats, *Mech. Ageing Dev.*, 57, 49, 1991.

68. Wirth, A. et al., Insulin kinetics and insulin binding to adipocytes in physically trained and food-restricted rats, *Am. J. Physiol.*, 238, E108, 1980.

69. Shimomura, I. et al., Marked reduction of acyl-CoA synthetase activity and messenger RNA in intra-abdominal visceral fat by physical exercise, *Am. J. Physiol.*, 265, E44, 1993.

70. Stallknecht, B. et al., The effect of lesions of the sympathoadrenal system on training-induced adaptations in adipocytes and pancreatic islets in rats, *Acta Physiol. Scand.*, 156, 465, 1996.

71. Ferrara, C.M. et al., Short-term exercise enhances insulin-stimulated GLUT-4 translocation and glucose transport in adipose cells, *J. Appl. Physiol.*, 85, 2106, 1998.

72. Viru, A., Toode, K., and Eller, A., Adipocyte responses to adrenaline and insulin in active and former sportsmen, *Eur. J. Appl. Physiol.*, 64, 345, 1992.

73. Savard, R. et al., Adipose tissue lipid accumulation pathways in marathon runners, *Int. J. Sports Med.*, 6, 287, 1985.

74. Poehlman, E.T. et al., Heredity and changes in body composition and adipose tissue metabolism after short-term exercise-training, *Eur. J. Appl. Physiol.*, 56, 398, 1987.

75. Savard, R. et al., Endurance training and glucose conversion into triglycerides in human fat cells, *J. Appl. Physiol.*, 58, 230, 1985.

76. Krotkiewski, M. et al., The effects of physical training on insulin secretion and effectiveness and on glucose metabolism in obesity and type 2 (non-insulin-dependent) diabetes mellitus, *Diabetologia*, 28, 881, 1985.

77. Rodnick, K.J. et al., Improved insulin action in muscle, liver, and adipose tissue in physically trained human subjects, *Am. J. Physiol.*, 253, E489, 1987.

78. James, D.E., Kraegen, E.W., and Chisholm, D.J., Effects of exercise training on in vivo insulin action in individual tissues of the rat, *J. Clin. Invest.*, 76, 657, 1985.

79. Enevoldsen, L.H. et al., Effect of exercise training on in vivo insulin-stimulated glucose uptake in intra-abdominal adipose tissue in rats, *Am. J. Physiol. Endocrinol. Metab.*, 278, E25, 2000.

80. Yang, W.P. et al., Effect of daily voluntary running on in vivo insulin action in rat skeletal muscle and adipose tissue as determined by the microdialysis technique, *Int. J. Sports Med.*, 16, 99, 1995.

81. Stallknecht, B. et al., Effect of training on insulin sensitivity of glucose uptake and lipolysis in human adipose tissue, *Am. J. Physiol. Endocrinol. Metab.*, 279, E376, 2000.

82. Foley, J.E., Foley, R., and Gliemann, J., Rate-limiting steps of 2-deoxyglucose uptake in rat adipocytes, *Biochim. Biophys. Acta,* 599, 689, 1980.
83. Martin, S., Slot, J.W., and James, D.E., GLUT4 trafficking in insulin-sensitive cells. A morphological review, *Cell Biochem. Biophys.,* 30, 89, 1999.
84. Cushman, S.W. and Wardzala, L.J., Potential mechanism of insulin action on glucose transport in the isolated rat adipose cell. Apparent translocation of intracellular transport systems to the plasma membrane, *J. Biol. Chem.,* 255, 4758, 1980.
85. Li, W.M. and McNeill, J.H., Quantitative methods for measuring the insulin-regulatable glucose transporter (GLUT4), *J. Pharmacol. Toxicol. Meth.,* 38, 1, 1997.
86. Kahn, B.B. and Flier, J.S., Regulation of glucose-transporter gene expression in vitro and in vivo, *Diabetes Care,* 13, 548, 1990.
87. Joost, H.G. and Weber, T.M., The regulation of glucose transport in insulin-sensitive cells, *Diabetologia,* 32, 831, 1989.
88. Ikemoto, S. et al., Expression of an insulin-responsive glucose transporter (GLUT4) minigene in transgenic mice: effect of exercise and role in glucose homeostasis, *Proc. Natl. Acad. Sci. USA,* 92, 865, 1995.
89. Coppack, S.W. et al., Carbohydrate metabolism in human adipose tissue in vivo, *Biochem. Soc. Trans.,* 17, 145, 1989.
90. Jansson, P.A., Smith, U., and Lönnroth, P., Evidence for lactate production by human adipose tissue in vivo, *Diabetologia,* 33, 253, 1990.
91. DeFronzo, R.A. et al., The effect of insulin on the disposal of intravenous glucose. Results from indirect calorimetry and hepatic and femoral venous catheterization, *Diabetes,* 30, 1000, 1981.
92. Mikines, K.J. et al., Effect of training on the dose-response relationship for insulin action in men, *J. Appl. Physiol.,* 66, 695, 1989.
93. Oshida, Y. et al., Effects of training and training cessation on insulin action, *Int. J. Sports Med.,* 12, 484, 1991.
94. Dela, F. et al., Effect of training on insulin-mediated glucose uptake in human muscle, *Am. J. Physiol.,* 263, E1134, 1992.

*chapter five*

# Exercise and adipose tissue production of cytokines

*Matthew S. Hickey and Richard G. Israel*

## Contents

## Dedication

This work is dedicated to the memory of Amy Paige Hickey (November 13, 1968–July 22, 2000) and to the future of our daughter, Meghan Elizabeth Hickey.

## 5.1  Background

Our understanding of the integrative biology of adipose tissue has changed dramatically in the half century since the publication of the classic review by Wertheimer and Shapiro,[1] which has aptly been described as "the beginning of the modern era in adipose tissue biology."[2] Wertheimer and Shapiro were the first to propose that adipose tissue is metabolically active and regulated by nervous and endocrine factors. Work in labs around the world has provided ample confirmation of this proposal, and the decades following this classic review were largely characterized by work describing adipocyte isolation procedures and the attendant study of the mechanisms of lipid synthesis, lipolysis, and insulin action.[2]

The recent explosion of interest in adipose tissue biology has been driven by an increasing appreciation of the role of adipose tissue as an endocrine organ that has the ability to influence organismal energy balance and nutrient partitioning.[3-13] In a 1990 review, Hollenberg[2] accurately predicted in a superb "state-of-the-art" review that the future of adipose tissue biology would focus on two main areas: (1) secretory products and (2) regulation of gene expression. Elegant work conducted in the last decade has provided a wealth of evidence documenting the remarkable complexity of adipose tissue biology. In addition to the canonical role of adipose tissue as a site for the storage and release of triacylglycerol,[1,2] we now know that this tissue synthesizes and secretes a large number of molecules (see Figure 5.1) involved in such diverse actions as lipid/cholesterol metabolism,[14-16] fibrinolysis,[17,18] immune function,[19-24] central regulation of ingestive behavior and energy expenditure,[25,26] insulin action,[27-40] and nutrient partitioning.[8] These secretory products can variously act in endocrine, autocrine, and paracrine fashion.[41] The pace of research in this discipline, the magnitude of interdisciplinary interest, and the growing list of biological systems/target tissues influenced by adipose tissue strongly suggest that the list of secretory products and biological functions of adipose tissue will continue to grow.

Because of the scope of this topic, this chapter will be limited to the discussion of two members of the cytokine family that are secreted by adipose tissue: the proinflammatory cytokine tumor necrosis factor-alpha (TNF-α) and the novel cytokine leptin, which is the product of the *obese* gene. Cytokine is derived from the Greek root meaning "to set cells in motion," [42] which is a highly appropriate description of the actions of these two molecules. Discussion of both TNF-α and leptin will include a brief history and overview of the molecular biology of these cytokines, followed by the consideration of how exercise may alter their secretion.

## 5.2   Tumor necrosis factor-alpha (TNF-α)

### 5.2.1   Historical perspective

Although TNF-α was isolated in 1984, suggestions in the medical literature of the presence of a secreted product that induced hemorrhagic necrosis in solid tumors date back over a century.[43] TNF-α is secreted from a variety of tissues including neutrophils, activated lymphocytes, macrophages,

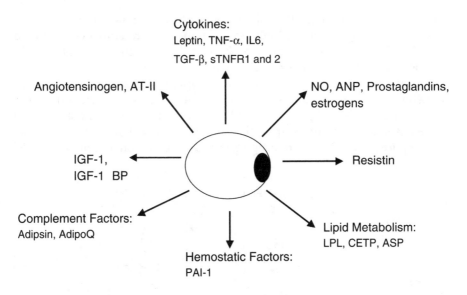

*Figure 5.1*    Secretory products of adipose tissue. IL6 = interleukin-6, TGF-$\beta$ = transforming growth factor-$\beta$, sTNFR = soluble form of the two TNF receptors. NO = nitric oxide; white adipose tissue expresses inducible nitric oxide synthase (iNOS). ANP = atrial natriuretic peptide. Resistin is a novel secreted factor from adipose tissue that is involved in regulating insulin action.[27] LPL = lipoprotein lipase, CETP = cholesterol ester transfer protein, ASP = acylation stimulating protein, PAI-1 = plasminogen activator inhibitor-1.

astrocytes, endothelial cells, smooth muscle cells, and white adipocytes.[43] In addition, there is good evidence that TNF-$\alpha$ is produced in skeletal muscle.[44] TNF-$\alpha$ was isolated independently by two labs and termed "cachectin" (from *cachexia*, or wasting) and "tumor necrosis factor."[43] It was subsequently confirmed that these proteins were identical.[45] Although much of the work investigating the biology of TNF-$\alpha$ has addressed its role as a proinflammatory cytokine, it is now clear that TNF-$\alpha$ has pleiotropic effects on a number of target tissues.[46]

## 5.2.2    Molecular biology

Tumor necrosis factor-$\alpha$ is produced as a biologically active 26-kDa membrane-bound monomer, or a secreted timer of 17-kDa subunits.[46] TNF-$\alpha$ is the product of a single gene located on chromosome 6 within the major histocompatibility complex.[46] All target tissues coexpress two receptor isoforms in varying ratios. These receptors are 60 and 80 kDa in humans (p60 and p80, or TNFR1 and TNFR2, respectively) and 55 and 75 kDa in other species (p55 and p75).[46] Membrane-bound receptors are homodimers of p60 or p80, and soluble forms of both receptor isoforms exist (following proteolytic cleavage of the extracellular domain).[46] Binding of TNF-$\alpha$ to either soluble receptor (sTNFR1 or 2) modulates the interaction with membrane-bound receptors and can accordingly regulate biological activity. It has recently been reported that sTNFR2 is increased in human obesity,[47–49] although the specific implications of this observation are not yet clear.

Tumor necrosis factor-α acts in an autocrine/paracine fashion in adipose tissue and has a wide variety of effects on adipose tissue metabolism and gene expression (see Figure 5.2). In addition to impairing insulin action and lipogenesis, TNF-α induces lipolysis (and, potentially, delipidation) and has been reported to induce both adipocyte dedifferentiation and apoptosis.[50,51]

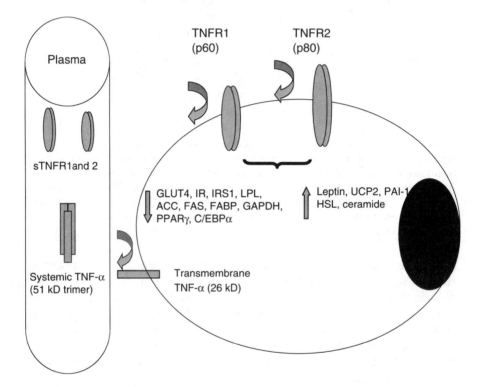

***Figure 5.2*** Overview of TNF-α and TNF-α receptor function. TNF-α is synthesized as a 26-kDa transmembrane protein. The transmembrane form is thought to have biological activity. Transmembrane TNF-α is proteolytically cleaved (arrow) to yield systemic TNF-α (a trimer of 17 kDa subunits). Both TNF receptors can also be proteolytically cleaved to yield soluble receptors (sTNFR1 and 2) that can bind TNF-α in circulation. GLUT4 = insulin-responsive glucose transporter, IR = insulin receptor, IRS1 = insulin receptor substrate 1, ACC = acetyl CoA carboxylase, FAS = fatty acid synthase, FABP = fatty acid binding protein, GAPDH = glyceraldehyde 3-phosphate dehydrogenase, PPARγ = peroxisome proliferator activated receptor γ, C/EBPα = CCAAT/enhancer binding protein alpha, UCP2 = uncoupling protein 2, PAI-1 = plasminogen activator inhibitor-1, HSL = hormone-sensitive lipase.

## 5.2.3 TNF-α response to exercise

Considerable controversy surrounds the effect of acute or chronic exercise on adipose tissue release of TNF-α.[52,53] It should be made clear that TNF-α generally circulates in extremely low concentrations and is often undetectable systemically.[53] Thus, apparent "systemic" effects (i.e., those on skeletal muscle) may be mediated by local production of TNF-α by skeletal muscle[44] or neighboring adipocytes or immune cells. Given the foregoing, several authors have urged caution in interpreting the existing data because the presence or absence of a change in *systemic* TNF-α is not likely to fully characterize the response of this cytokine to exercise.[52,53] Further, it must be made clear that the presence or absence of systemic changes in TNF-α following exercise does *not* imply that adipocytes are responsive/nonresponsive; that is, in the absence of exercise-induced changes in *plasma* TNF-α, one cannot exclude autocrine/paracrine effects of this cytokine within an adipose tissue depot that may have significant biological effects. Moreover, in cases where systemic elevations in TNF-α have been observed, the source is not necessarily adipose tissue. These important considerations must be kept in mind when interpreting the data in this area.

Early work by Cannon and associates[54] highlighted the challenge of studying TNF-α responses to even very strenuous exercise. These authors reported on both plasma concentration of TNF-α and *in vitro* endotoxin (lipopolysaccharide, or LPS)-induced production of TNF-α, from isolated mononuclear cells, following downhill running. The exercise consisted of three 15-min bouts of downhill running (−16%) at an intensity equivalent to 75% of maximal heart rate. Twenty-four hours after exercise, *in vitro* LPS-induced TNF-α production was increased by 60%.[54] In contrast, plasma TNF-α peaked at 6 hr post-exercise and was nearly undetectable at 24 hr post-exercise.[54] Importantly, even at 6 hr post-exercise, only 5 of 14 subjects had detectable levels of TNF-α. Further, the median plasma TNF-α 6 hr post-exercise was <10 pg/mL, whereas the same group has reported plasma concentrations of 110 and 890 pg/mL in septic shock and endotoxin infusion, respectively.[54]

Early work by Espersen and colleagues[55] reported an increase in plasma TNF-α following both a 2.5-hr run and a 5-km race. Although the majority of subsequent work failed to confirm these observations,[56–60] recent work by Ostrowski et al.[61] has provided evidence of a twofold increase in plasma TNF-α following the 1997 Copenhagen Marathon. Importantly, these authors also observed approximately twofold increases in the plasma concentration of *both* soluble TNF-α receptor isoforms,[61] which may have limited the bioavailability of TNF-α.

In contrast to the foregoing observations, the same group has studied exercise-induced increases in plasma cytokines following a 2.5-hr treadmill run at 75% $VO_2$max. Blood was sampled before exercise, every 30 min during exercise, and every hour during a 6-hr recovery period. Under these circumstances, no change in plasma TNF-α was detected (despite increases in IL-6 and IL-1ra).[62] Similarly, Suzuki et al.[63] recently reported the cytokine response to a marathon run in 16 male subjects. Plasma TNF-α was unde-tectable in baseline samples obtained the day prior to the race or in imme-diate post-race samples.

The underlying reasons for the discrepancies in the literature are not clear, although Camus et al.[64] have recently suggested that exercise-induced changes in plasma TNF-α may require a transient endotoxemia. Exercise-induced endotoxemia is poorly understood but is thought to result from changes in intestinal permeability secondary to reduced splanchnic blood flow, dehydration, and hyperthermia.[64] Camus et al.[64] studied 14 male tri-athletes before and after a competition (1.5-km swim, 40-km bike, 10-km run; mean time 149.8 ± 4.8 min). Plasma TNF-α concentrations increased from 18.0 ± 1.5 pg/mL prior to the race to a peak of 31.0 ± 1.8 pg/mL 1 hr post-race. The race was associated with a transient endotoxemia, as evi-denced by changes in several anti-LPS IgG and IgM activities. The authors suggest that at least some of the discordant results in the literature may be related to the absence of endotoxemia in some of the studies with negative results. Although this may be the case, it is important to bear in mind that a number of studies utilizing prolonged, strenuous exercise have failed to report changes in plasma TNF-α, despite conditions that were likely to have induced the changes in intestinal blood flow, hydration, and thermoregula-tion postulated to increase intestinal permeability.[57–60] Alternatively, endot-oxin tolerance subsequent to repeated exposure has been reported,[64] and it is possible that training state (and the degree of habitual exposure to exercise-induced endotoxemia) could minimize changes in TNF-α. It should be noted that several groups have reported that prior exercise inhibits *ex vivo* LPS-induced TNF-α secretion,[56,57] an effect that may be mediated by inhibi-tion of TNF-α release by cortisol.[65]

## 5.2.4   Summary

What is clear from the foregoing is that the plasma TNF-α response to exercise is controversial. Moreover, very little research has investigated local changes in adipose tissue production of this cytokine — research that may help clarify what role, if any, TNF-α may play in exercise metabolism. Although the study of potential autocrine/paracrine effects is clearly more difficult than assessing systemic changes, it would appear that designs uti-lizing adipose tissue microdialysis may help address this question. One group has recently utilized A-V balance techniques to study release of TNF-α from subcutaneous adipose tissue.[66] Thirty-nine subjects with a mean body mass index (BMI) of 31.8 kg/m² were studied in a resting, post-absorptive state. No adipose tissue production of TNF-α was observed under these conditions, despite a twofold A-V difference in IL-6. Of course, the absence of basal TNF-α release does not preclude subcutaneous adipose tissue from producing substantial amounts of TNF-α during periods of physiological stress. In addition to the need for further work characterizing local adipose tissue TNF-α production, more work is needed to clarify the biological role of local or systemic changes in this potent hormone.

## 5.3   Leptin

### 5.3.1   Historical perspective

The cloning of the murine obese gene and its human homolog in 1994 by Friedman's group[67] was a watershed in adipose tissue biology. In addition to highlighting a rich chapter in the history of physiology by providing evidence that the lipostatic factor postulated from the work of Kennedy[68] nearly 40 years earlier had been discovered, the discovery of leptin stimulated tremendous interdisciplinary interest in the study of adipose tissue biology in the context of its role as an endocrine regulator of energy balance. The study history of the obese (ob/ob) mouse is a rich one and includes some remarkably elegant work utilizing parabiosis to study integrative physiology.[69] Interestingly, both the phenotypic characteristics of the ob/ob mouse as well as the chromosomal location of the affected gene were known for several decades before the cloning of leptin.[70] We now know that ob/ob mice do not produce a functional form of leptin and as a result are massively obese. Not long after the report of the cloning of the obese gene, three independent labs reported the first results of recombinant leptin administration on ob/ob mice,[71–73] and the results were rather striking: Leptin administration resulted in reduced food intake, increased body temperature, increased oxygen consumption, and selective loss of body fat. These studies provided unequivocal evidence of the biological activity of leptin in this rodent model of obesity. The interest generated by the cloning of the *obese* gene and the initial reports of potent biological activity is best appreciated by the pace of research in this area. In the 5-year period since the cloning was reported, over 3000 peer-reviewed scholarly publications have addressed various aspects of leptin biology in rodents and humans. This is a remarkable pace of research and reflects strong interdisciplinary interest in the pathogenesis of obesity.

### 5.3.2   Molecular biology

Leptin is a peptide of 146 amino acids that circulates as a 16-kDa monomer[9] in both bound and free forms.[9] Leptin is expressed in and secreted primarily from white adipose tissue,[9] although evidence indicates that it may also be produced by skeletal muscle,[74] gastric epithelial cells,[75] brain,[76,77] and the placenta.[78] The quantitative contribution of these other sites of leptin production to systemic leptin concentration is not clear.

Leptin receptors belong to the class I cytokine receptor family,[9,79] which signals intracellularly through the JAK–STAT pathway.[9] A number of splice variants of the leptin receptor exist, with tissue-specific expression patterns. Leptin receptors are expressed in a variety of tissues, including the hypothalamus, choroids plexus, β cells of the pancreas, adipose tissue, liver, kidney, jejunum, lung, adrenal medulla, ovaries, testes, placenta, heart, and skeletal muscle.[9,79] The long form of the leptin receptor, termed OB-Rb, is preferentially expressed in the hypothalamus and is the most thoroughly studied to date. Evidence from the study of obese db/db mice, which are unresponsive to leptin, provides convincing evidence that OB-Rb is required for the action of leptin on food intake and energy expenditure.[6,8–10,13] The db/db mice have a mutation that leads to the production of a truncated form of OB-Rb.[9,77] The predominant short form of the receptor, OB-Ra, is expressed in a number of peripheral tissues and in the choroids plexus.[9] Ob-Re, another short form of the receptor, is thought to be a soluble form of the receptor and may act as a binding protein (see Figure 5.3).[9]

Leptin action at target tissues can include both changes in gene expression and intermediary metabolism (see Figure 5.4). What has emerged from 5 years of intense study of leptin secretion and action is that leptin is not simply an "anti-obesity" hormone, nor does it always reflect adipose tissue mass. In fact, it has been suggested that leptin is primarily an anti-starvation

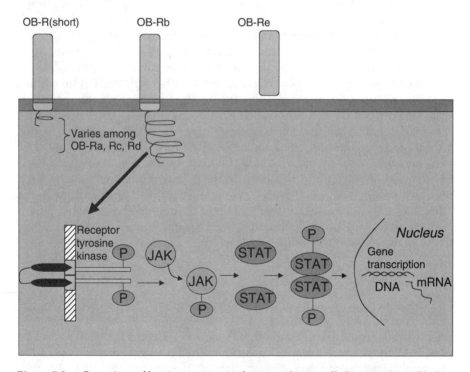

*Figure 5.3*    Overview of leptin receptor isoforms and intracellular signaling. Ob-Ra, -Rc, and -Rd all have short cytoplasmic domains; Ob-Rb is the full-length receptor and a complete cytoplasmic domain and signals through the JAK (janus kinase)–STAT (signal transducers and effectors of transcription) pathway. Ob-Re is a soluble form of the leptin receptor.

hormone.[3,80] The response of systemic leptin to partial or total energy restriction is a rapid and profound decrease, implying that energy restriction is a potent signal to reduce leptin secretion. Leptin appears to be involved in regulating the physiological adjustments to starvation,[80] which defend the organism from excess energy expenditure in the face of limited availability of energy intake. From a survival standpoint, regulating this response is likely to be much more relevant than defending against excess accumulation of body fat (at least until recently).[3] In addition to the role of leptin in defending the organism against starvation, Unger and associates[81] have recently postulated that a primary function of leptin is to regulate the triglyceride content in cells *other than* adipocytes. This hypothesis suggests that leptin serves to maintain triglyceride content within a narrow range in non-adipocytes to avoid lipotoxicity. Because adipocytes have a virtually unlimited capacity to store triglyceride, the action of leptin to partition nutrients toward adipose tissue serves as a "defense" mechanism to maintain the viability and function of other tissues that have a limited functional triglyceride storage capacity.[81]

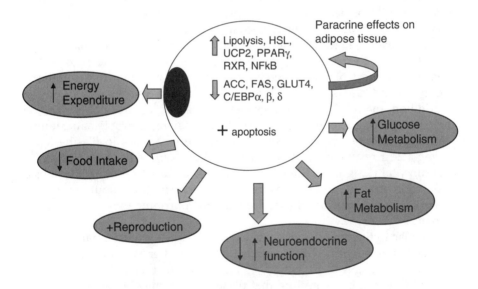

*Figure 5.4*   General actions of leptin. Systemic leptin can act upon a number of target tissues to effect changes in energy expenditure and energy intake, and reproductive and neuroendocrine function, as well as to alter lipid and glucose metabolism. In addition, leptin has autocrine/paracrine actions on adipose tissue function that can include upregulation of lipolysis and induction of HSL (hormone-sensitive lipase), UCP2 (uncoupling protein 2), PPARγ (peroxisome proliferator activated receptor γ), RXR (the retinoid X receptor), and NFκB (nuclear factor κB). Also, leptin can downregulate the expression of ACC (acetyl CoA carboxylase), FAS (fatty acid synthase), GLUT4, and C/EBP (CCAAT/enhancer binding protein) isoforms. Leptin has also been shown to induce apoptosis in white adipocytes.

### 5.3.3   Effect of exercise on adipose tissue leptin secretion

The physiological stress of exercise is an obvious potential regulator of leptin secretion by adipose tissue. The attendant changes in fuel flux, systemic hormone concentrations, and energy expenditure may influence plasma leptin concentration, and presumably, leptin action. Interestingly, despite the rather remarkable pace of research on leptin, less than three dozen studies have specifically addressed exercise–leptin interactions in humans. Although space limitations preclude a detailed discussion of all the work in this area, research on leptin and exercise has in general taken three traditional approaches: cross-sectional studies, acute (single-bout) exercise studies, and exercise training. Studies investigating large databases have in general reported that the log of plasma leptin is inversely related to "fitness" (maximal treadmill time, $VO_2$max),[82–84] but this relationship is generally not independent of adiposity. In contrast, some studies with discrete groups of athletes vs. sedentary controls have suggested an effect of chronic exercise training that could not be entirely accounted for by differences in fat mass.[85,86] The implication from these studies is that some aspect of habitual physical training may specifically reduce systemic leptin concentration (i.e., beyond what can be explained by the lower fat mass in athletes).

Acute exercise studies have generally shown no effect on plasma leptin,[87–93] unless the energy expenditure is profound.[94–96] The studies that reported an effect of acute exercise have generally shown that significant energy expenditure is required before systemic leptin is affected by exercise. In addition, many of these studies lacked a resting control period, and, as such, interpreting apparent exercise-induced changes is problematic. Importantly, Landt et al.[94] reported similar magnitude changes in plasma leptin during a 2-hr resting control period and a 2-hr exercise bout. Differences in experimental design, including the nature of the exercise bout, the subject population studied, and the relative lack of information about any energy intake during the period of exercise may all contribute to some of the discrepancies reported.

Similar to the majority of acute exercise studies, exercise training interventions have suggested that exercise does not alter systemic leptin independent of changes in fat mass.[97–101] Exceptions to this include work from the author's group, suggesting that plasma leptin may be reduced in exercise-trained females (but not males in an identical training program) despite stable fat mass,[102] and a study from Saris's group suggesting that an independent effect of exercise on plasma leptin is detectable after 10 months of training.[103] It is important to note, however, that in general neither the acute exercise studies nor the training interventions controlled for energy balance, and most sampled only a single fasting plasma leptin pre- and post-intervention. Two recent studies have elegantly demonstrated the care that is necessary to study leptin–exercise interactions.[104,105] Because leptin is acutely sensitive to negative energy balance (fasting or caloric restriction), it is important to design studies that can distinguish the effects of exercise per se from any attendant change in energy balance or, perhaps more specifically, energy availability (see Figure 5.5). Moreover, leptin, like many other hormones, exhibits a clear diurnal rhythm.[6,9,12] Because the vast majority of research on exercise to date has incorporated only a single fasting sample, drawing conclusions from this "snapshot" of the diurnal pattern is difficult. The characterization of 24-hr plasma leptin profiles provides a much more informative (and representative) view of the dynamic effects of exercise on leptin.

Van Aggel-Leijssen et al.[104] studied eight healthy, lean (14.5% fat), sedentary males under four conditions: (1) no exercise–energy balance, (2) exercise–energy balance (2-hr exercise at 50% VO$_2$max, equivalent to ~800 kcal),

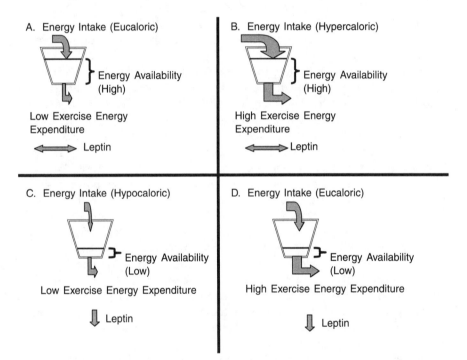

*Figure 5.5* The energy availability hypothesis. Energy availability is operationally defined as energy intake minus exercise energy expenditure. Panel A depicts a eucaloric diet and low or no exercise condition. Energy availability is high, and plasma leptin is unaffected. Panel B depicts a condition in which exercise energy expenditure is high and energy intake is high, resulting in the maintenance of high-energy availability. In this scenario, despite the exercise, plasma leptin is unaffected. Panel C depicts a low-energy diet and low or no exercise. Despite the small amount of activity-related energy expenditure, energy availability is low, and plasma leptin decreases. Panel D depicts a eucaloric diet combined with a high exercise–energy expenditure, resulting in low energy availability and a reduction in plasma leptin. This schematic is based on the experimental design and energy availability hypothesis of Hilton and Loucks.[105] It is important to note that this study measured 24-hr leptin rhythms and not a single fasting sample.

(3) exercise–negative energy balance (energy deficit of ~800 kcal), and (4) exercise–positive energy balance (energy surplus of ~833 kcal). Interestingly, the exercise–energy balance condition resulted in a 20% reduction in the weighted average 24-hr leptin concentration. In contrast, the exercise–negative energy balance condition, which is considered a greater energetic stressor, did not alter 24-hr leptin concentration. This is paradoxical in the sense that the exercise energy expenditure was matched in both conditions, but it was the condition in which subjects were fed to achieve energy balance that average 24-hr leptin was reduced. One obvious conclusion is that some aspect of the feeding resulted in the reduced leptin in the exercise–energy balance trial, which is also difficult to conceptualize. The exercise–positive energy balance condition did not alter average 24-hr leptin concentration but did increase the amplitude of the 24-hr leptin curve by twofold compared with the exercise–energy balance condition.

It is also important to note that no treatment altered baseline (9:00 a.m.) plasma leptin concentration in this study, reinforcing the view that the earlier studies were correct to this extent but likely missed effects of the exercise bout on 24-hr leptin profiles by studying only a single fasting plasma sample. Finally, it should be noted that stepwise regression analysis suggested that 98% of the variance in 24-hr plasma leptin could be explained by the combination of fasting plasma nonesterified fatty acids and glucose. Although this may be taken as indirect support of the concept that leptin expression is regulated by some aspect of fuel flux in adipose tissue,[74,106] the cellular mechanisms of such a regulatory pathway(s) remain incompletely understood.

Hilton and Loucks[105] incorporated a similar design to study the influence of energy availability on 24-hr average leptin concentration. Energy availability was operationally defined in this study as the difference between dietary energy intake and controlled exercise energy expenditure (energy intake – exercise energy expenditure = energy availability). Put another way, energy availability is the amount of dietary energy "left over" for other biological processes after exercise had consumed a given amount of the daily energy budget (see Figure 5.5).

Sixteen healthy, eumenorrheic women were studied. Subjects were assigned to either non-exercise or exercise groups and each group was then studied twice. The no-exercise group completed two trials:

1.   *Balanced-energy availability* (both energy intake and energy availability = 45 kcal/kg lean body mass or LBM/day, equivalent to a habitual energy intake of ~2000 kcal/day in these subjects).
2.   *Low-energy availability* (energy intake and energy availability = 10 kcal/kg LBM/day, equivalent to 78% energy restriction, or ~430 kcal/day).

Energy availability in the exercise group was matched to the sedentary subjects (i.e., energy availability = 45 kcal/kg LBM/day in the balanced-energy trial and 10 kcal/kg LBM/day in the low-energy trial). The matching was achieved by fixing exercise energy expenditure at 30 kcal/kg LBM/day in both exercise trials (~1300 kcal/day) and varying energy intake accordingly. An important difference from van Aggel-Leijssen et al.[104] is that each diet or diet-plus-exercise treatment lasted 4 days.

When energy availability was matched between groups, exercise was without effect on either the 24-hr mean or the amplitude of the diurnal leptin rhythm. In contrast, irrespective of the magnitude of exercise energy expenditure, low-energy availability reduced both the 24-hr mean (–72%, –53%) and amplitude (–85%, –58%) of the diurnal leptin rhythm for the no-exercise and exercise groups, respectively. It is important to note that the reductions in leptin in the exercise group occurred during a 4-day period when total energy intake in this group was ~1700 kcal. Thus, an important observation from this study is that leptin responds not to energy intake (or expenditure) per se but acts as a sensor of the *difference* between energy intake and expenditure.[105]

The cellular mechanism(s) by which leptin responds to differences between energy intake and expenditure is not clearly understood at this time. Hilton and Loucks[105] suggest that leptin may in fact be responding to changes in carbohydrate availability, and several other groups have provided evidence that intracellular products of glucose metabolism in the hexosamine pathway are involved in regulating leptin secretion.[74,106] If further work confirms that a product of hexosamine metabolism acts as a regulator of leptin secretion, then the "lipostat" may in fact be regulated more closely by what may be considered "glucostatic" factors (see Figure 5.6).

Key differences in the experimental design in the studies by van Aggel-Leijssen et al. and Hilton and Loucks should be noted. The low-energy availability condition of Hilton and Loucks represented a 78% reduction in habitual energy intake for a period of 4 days. Although there is no directly comparable condition in the study of van Aggel-Leijssen et al., the exercise–negative energy balance (28% negative energy for 24 hr) condition in this study was without effect on the 24-hr mean and amplitude of the diurnal leptin rhythm. As Hilton and Loucks suggest, this would imply a threshold reduction in energy availability that must be reached to alter the dynamics of the diurnal rhythm of leptin, or there may be a gender difference in the sensitivity of leptin to changes in energy availability. It is also possible that the moderate negative energy balance of –28% would require more than 24 hr to impact the leptin rhythm.

### 5.3.4 Summary

The work of van Aggel-Leijssen et al. and Hilton and Loucks is both elegant and informative. The studies are useful in that they provide evidence of the limitation of studies using a single fasting blood sample to assess diet/exercise effects on systemic leptin. Both studies also make it clear that careful consideration of energy balance is warranted when studying the biology of leptin. Because of the differences in gender and design between these studies,

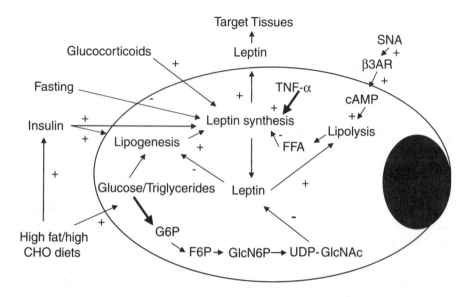

*Figure 5.6* Overview of the regulation of leptin secretion from white adipose tissue. SNA = sympathetic nervous system activation, β3AR = β3 adrenergic receptor. The pathway of G6P (= glucose 6-phosphate), F6P (= fructose 6-phosphate), GlcN6Pm (= glucosamine 6-phosphate), UDP-GlcNAC (= UDP-*N*-acetylglucosamine) represents steps in the hexosamine biosynthesis pathway that have been implicated in leptin gene expression. (Data from Wang, J. et al., *Nature*, 393, 684, 1998.)

generalizations about the effect of exercise on leptin remain elusive. However, should the work of Hilton and Loucks be confirmed (particularly in males), it will provide additional support for the hypothesis that leptin responds not to energy intake or exercise energy expenditure alone, but to the balance between the two. Because recent evidence suggests that 24-hr leptin levels may predict subsequent food intake,[107] exercise-induced alterations in the 24-hr leptin rhythm can impact the regulation of energy balance in the organism over a period of days.

The fact that leptin may not respond to isolated components of energy balance (i.e., intake or expenditure alone) is perhaps not surprising. The ability of an organism to "sense" both the energy expenditure and energy requirements is essential to appropriately respond to both energy deficits and energy surplus. The maintenance of an appropriate energy budget on a day-to-day basis, when energy expended in physical activity, total energy expenditure, and energy intake may all be changing, is obviously an essential component of both survival and viability.

It should be clear that much more work needs to be done regarding how exercise impacts leptin secretion, clearance, and, most important, leptin action at target tissues. Our understanding of the integrative biology of leptin has progressed considerably in the past 6 years. These continued research efforts have primarily served to highlight the complexity of the energy-balance regulatory systems.

## 5.4    Conclusions

Tumor necrosis factor-α and leptin, secretory products of adipose tissue and members of the cytokine superfamily, have been the focus of intense interest because of their diverse and often potent actions on intermediary metabolism at target tissues. Their role in exercise (or recovery) metabolism is not clear at this point. It is safe to conclude that for both cytokines the stress of exercise must be rather pronounced in order to induce a systemic change in either hormone. In the case of TNF-α, recent studies have postulated that exercise-induced endotoxemia may be a "trigger" for increases in systemic concentration.[64] In this context, elevations in TNF-α may reflect more of a "canonical" role for this cytokine (i.e., immunomodulation) than a specific role in exercise metabolism. Recent work characterizing the 24-hr leptin response to manipulations of diet plus exercise has provided preliminary evidence that leptin responds not to exercise per se, but to energy availability. This is an intriguing concept that requires additional work.

In the few reports that document an exercise effect on TNF-α and leptin, the magnitude of change in both cases is rather modest: generally less than a twofold increase for TNF-α and less than a 50% decrease for leptin, even after extreme exercise. It is important to bear in mind that leptin expression can be regulated by TNF-α,[108,109] and, as such, interactions between these two cytokines may occur at the level of expression/secretion, in addition to potential interactions in terms of regulating metabolism at target tissues. Both TNF-α and leptin can be bound in circulation,[22,110] and it is unclear how exercise alters either the binding kinetics of either cytokine to soluble receptors.

Importantly, virtually no evidence about local changes in either cytokine exists that may be relevant in terms of autocrine or paracrine functions, which would be missed in designs that sample only systemic hormone concentrations. Despite the lack of convincing evidence to date that either hormone plays a substantive role in the physiological adjustments to exercise, the story is far from being fully told. Continued progress in both adipose tissue biology and on the endocrinology of exercise will undoubtedly shed additional light on these two profoundly interesting hormones.

## Acknowledgments

The assistance provided by Amanda Malek and Leah Nein in typesetting the manuscript is greatly appreciated. Comments provided by Dr. Tracy Nelson and Dr. Kevin Davy were invaluable. The authors also thank their colleagues at East Carolina University for their collaboration on these studies. In addition, the collaborative contributions of Dr. Jose Caro and Dr. Robert Considine made these studies possible.

# References

1. Wertheimer, E. and Shapiro, B., Physiology of adipose tissue, *Physiol. Rev.*, 28, 451, 1948.
2. Hollenberg, C.H., Perspectives in adipose tissue biology, *Int. J. Obesity*, 14(suppl. 3), 135, 1990.
3. Flier, J.S., What's in a name? In search of leptin's physiologic role, *J. Clin. Endocrinol. Metab.*, 83(5), 1407, 1998.
4. Thong, F.S. and Graham, T.E., Leptin and reproduction: is it a critical link between adipose tissue, nutrition, and reproduction? *Can. J. Appl. Physiol.*, 24(4), 317, 1999.
5. Fried, S.K. and Russell, C.D., Diverse roles of adipose tissue in the regulation of systemic metabolism and energy balance, in *Handbook of Obesity*, G.A. Bray, C. Bouchard, and W.P.T. James, Eds., Marcel-Dekker, New York, 1998, pp. 397–413.
6. Harris, R.B.S., Leptin: much more than a satiety signal, *Annu. Rev. Nutr.*, 20, 45, 2000.
7. Bray, G.A. and York, D.A., The Mona Lisa hypothesis in the time of leptin, *Recent Prog. Hormone Res.*, 53, 95, 1998.
8. Baile, C.A., Della-Fera, M.A., and Martin, R.J., Regulation of metabolism and body fat mass by leptin, *Annu. Rev. Nutr.*,, 20, 105, 2000.
9. Friedman, J.M. and Halaas, J.L., Leptin and the regulation of body weight in mammals, *Nature*, 395, 763, 1998.
10. Casanueva, F.F. and Dieguez, C., Neuroendocrine regulation and actions of leptin, *Frontiers Neuroendocrinol.*, 20, 317, 1999.
11. Coleman, R.A. and Herrmann, T.S., Nutritional regulation of leptin in humans, *Diabetologia*, 42, 639, 1999.
12. Considine, R.V. and Caro, J.F., Leptin and the regulation of body weight, *Int. J. Biochem. Cell Bio.*, 29, 12545, 1997.
13. Himms-Hagen, J., Physiological roles of the leptin endocrine system: differences between mice and humans, *Crit. Rev. Clin. Lab. Sci.*, 36(9), 575, 1999.
14. Maslowska, M., Cianflone, K., and Rosenbloom, M., Acylation stimulating protein (ASP): role in adipose tissue, in *Progress in Obesity Tesearch*, Vol. 8, B. Guy-Grand and G. Ailhaud, Eds. John Libbey & Co., New York, 1998, pp. 65–70.
15. Sengenès, C., Natriuretic peptides: a new lipolytic pathway in human adipocytes, *FASEB J.*, 14, 1345, 2000.
16. Cianflone, K., Maslowska, M., and Sniderman, A.D., Acylation stimulating protein (ASP), an adipocyte autocrine: new directions, *Cell Devel. Biol.*, 10, 31, 1999.
17. Crandall, D.L., Quinet, E.M., Morgan, G.A., Busler, D.E., McHendry-Rinde, B., and Kral, J.G., Synthesis and secretion of plasminogen activator inhibitor-1 by human preadipocytes, *J. Clin. Endocrinol. Metab.*, 84, 3222, 1999.
18. Cigolini, M., Tonoli, M., Borgato, L., Frigotto, L., Manzato, F., Zeminian, S., Cardinale, C., Camin, M., Chiaramonte, E., DeSandre, G., and Lunardi, C., Expression of plasminogen activator inhibitor-1 in human adipose tissue: a role for TNF-α? *Atherosclerosis*, 143, 81, 1999.
19. Bullo-Bonet, M., Garcia-Lorda, P., Lopez-Soriano, F.J., Argiles, J.M., and Salvas-Salvado, J., Tumor necrosis factor: a key role in obesity? *FEBS Lett.*, 451, 215, 1999.

20. Sethi, J.K. and Hotamisligil, G.S., The role of TNF-α in adipocyte metabolism, *Semin. Cell Dev. Biol.*, 10, 19, 1999.

21. Kirchgessner, T.G., Uysal, K.T., Wiesbrock, S.M., Marino, M.W., and Hotamisligil, G.S., Tumor necrosis factor-α contributes to obesity-related hyperleptinemia by regulating leptin release from adipocytes, *J. Clin. Invest.*, 100, 2777, 1997.

22. Hauner, H., Bender, M., Haastert, B., and Hube, F., Plasma concentrations of soluble TNF-α receptors in obese subjects, *Int. J. Obesity*, 22, 1239, 1998.

23. Argiles, J.M., Lopez-Soriano, J., Busquets, S., and Lopez-Soriano, F.J., Journey from cachexia to obesity by TNF, *FASEB J.*, 11, 743, 1997.

24. Mohamed-Ali, V., Goodrick, S., Rawesh, A., Katz, D.R., Miles J.M., Yudkin J.S., Klein S., and Coppack, S.W., Subcutaneous adipose tissue releases interleukin-6, but not tumor necrosis factor-alpha, in-vivo, *J. Clin. Endocrinol. Metab.*, 82(12), 4196, 1997.

25. Flier, J., The adipocyte: storage depot or node on the energy information superhighway? *Cell*, 80, 15, 1995.

26. Loftus, T.M., An adipocyte-central nervous system regulatory loop in the control of adipose homeostasis, *Cell Dev. Biol.*, 10, 11, 1999.

27. Steppan, C.M., Bailey, S.T., Bhat, S., Brown, E.J., Banerjee, R.R., Wright, C.M., Patel, H.R., Ahima, R.S., and Lazar, M.A., The hormone resistin links obesity to diabetes, *Nature*, 409, 307, 2001.

28. Uysal, K.T., Wiesbrock, S.M., Marino, M.W., and Hotamisligil, G.S., Protection from obesity-induced insulin resistance in mice lacking TNF-α function, *Nature*, 389, 610, 1997.

29. Ventre, J., Doebber, T., Wu, M., MacNaul, K., Stevens, K., Pasparakis, M., Kollias, G., and Moller, D.E., Targeted disruption of the tumor necrosis factor-α gene. Metabolic consequences in obese and nonobese mice, *Diabetes*, 46, 1526, 1997.

30. Lofgren, P., van Harmelen, V., Reynisdottir, S., Naslund, E., Ryden, M., Rossner, S., and Arner, P., Secretion of tumor necrosis factor-alpha shows a strong relationship to insulin-stimulated glucose transport in human adipose tissue, *Diabetes*, 49(5), 688, 2000.

31. Moller, D.E., Potential role of TNF-α in the pathogenesis of insulin resistance and type 2 diabetes, *Trends Endocrinol. Metab.*, 11(6), 212, 2000.

32. Kern, P.A., Saghizadeh, M., Ong, J.M., Bosch, R.J., Deem, R., and Simsolo, R.B. The expression of tumor necrosis factor in human adipose tissue: regulation by obesity, weight loss, and relationship to lipoprotein lipase, *J. Clin. Invest.*, 95, 2111, 1995.

33. Hotamisligil, G.S., Shargill, N.S., and Speigelman, B.M., Adipose expression of tumor necrosis factor-alpha: direct role in obesity-linked insulin resistance, *Science*, 259, 87, 1993.

34. Hotamisligil, G.S., Arner, P., Caro, J.F., Atkinson, R.L., and Spiegelman, B.L., Increased adipose tissue expression of tumor necrosis factor-alpha in human obesity and insulin resistance, *J. Clin. Invest.*, 95, 2409, 1995.

35. Hotamisligil, G.S., Murray, D.L., Choy, L.N., and Spiegelman, B.L., Tumor necrosis factor-α inhibits signaling from the insulin receptor, *Proc. Natl. Acad. Sci. USA*, 91, 4854, 1994.

36. Feinstein, R., Kanety, H., Papa, M.Z., Lunefeld, B., and Karasik, A., Tumor necrosis factor-α suppresses insulin-induced tyrosine phosphorylation of insulin receptor and its substrates, *J. Biol. Chem.*, 268, 26055, 1993.

37. Hotamisligil, G.S., Peraldi, P., Budaveri, A., Ellis, R., White, M.F., and Spiegelman, B.L., IRS-1-mediated inhibition of insulin receptor tyrosine kinase activity in TNF-α and obesity-induced insulin resistance, *Science*, 271, 665, 1996.

38. Peraldi, P., Hotamisligil, G.S., Buurman, W.A., White, M.F., and Spiegelman, B.L., Tumor necrosis factor (TNF)-α inhibits insulin signaling through stimulation of p55TNF receptor and activation of sphingomyelinase, *J. Biol. Chem.*, 271, 13018, 1996.

39. Fernandez-Real, J.M., Gutierrez, C., Ricart, W., Casamitjana, R., Fernandez-Castaner, M., Vendrell, J., Richart, C., and Soler, J. The TNF-α NCO I polymorphism influences the relationship among insulin resistance, percent body fat, and increased serum leptin levels, *Diabetes*, 46, 1468, 1997.

40. Ofei, F., Hurel, S., Newkirk, J., Sopwith, M., and Taylor R., Effects of an engineered human anti-TNF-α antibody (CDP571) on insulin sensitivity and glycemic control in patients with NIDDM, *Diabetes*, 45, 881, 1996.

41. Mohamed-Ali, V., Pinkney, J.H., and Coppack, S.W., Adipose tissue as an endocrine and paracrine organ, *Int. J. Obesity*, 22, 1145, 1998.

42. Cannon, J.G., Inflammatory cytokines in nonpathological states, *Newsl. Physiol. Sci.*, 15, 298, 2000.

43. Beutler, B. and Cerami, A., Tumor necrosis, cachexia, shock, and inflammation: a common mediator, *Ann. Rev. Biochem.*, 57, 505, 1988.

44. Saghizadeh, M., Ong, J.M., Garvey, W.T., Henry, R.R., and Kern, P.A. The expression of TNF-α by human muscle. Relationship to insulin resistance, *J. Clin. Invest.*, 97(4), 1111, 1996.

45. Beutler, B., Greenwald, D., Hulmes, J.D., Chang, M., Pan, Y.C., Mathison, J., Ulevitch, R., and Cerami, A., Identity of tumor necrosis factor and the macrophage secreted factor cachectin, *Nature*, 316, 552, 1985.

46. Hotamisligil, G.S. and Speigelman, B.M., TNF-α and the insulin resistance of obesity, in *Diabetes Mellitus: A Fundamental and Clinical Text*, D. LeRoith, S.I. Taylor, and J.M. Olefsky, Eds., Lippincott-Raven, Philadelphia, 1997, pp. 554–565.

47. Hotamisligil, G.S., Arner, P., Atkinson, R.L., and Spiegelman, B.L., Differential regulation of the p80 tumor necrosis factor receptor in human obesity and insulin resistance, *Diabetes*, 46, 451, 1997.

48. Chu, N.F., Spiegelman, D., Rifai, N., Hotamisligil, G.S., and Rimm, E.B., Glycemic status and soluble tumor necrosis factor receptor levels in relation to plasma leptin concentrations among normal weight and overweight U.S. men, *Int. J. Obesity*, 24(9), 1085, 2000.

49. Ronnemaa, T., Pulkki, K., and Kaprio, J., Serum tumor necrosis factor-alpha receptor 2 is elevated in obesity but is not related to insulin sensitivity: a study in identical twins discordant for obesity, *J. Clin. Endocrinol. Metab.*, 85(8), 2728, 2000.

50. Prins, J.B. and O'Rahilly, S., Regulation of adipose cell number in man, *Clin. Sci.*, 92, 3, 1997.

51. Prins, J.B., Niesler, C.U., Winterford, C.M., Bright, N.A., Siddle, K., O'Rahilly, S., Walker, N.I., and Cameron, D.P., Tumor necrosis factor-α induces apoptosis of human adipose cells, *Diabetes*, 46, 1939, 1997.

52. Halle, M., Berg, A., Northoff, H., and Keul, J., Importance of TNF-α and leptin in obesity and insulin resistance: a hypothesis on the impact of physical exercise, *Exerc. Immunol. Rev.*, 4, 77, 1998.

53. Pedersen, B.K., Ostrowksi, K., Rohde, T., and Bruunsgaard, H., The cytokine response to strenuous exercise, *Can. J. Physiol. Pharmacol.*, 76, 505, 1998.
54. Cannon, J.G., Meydani, S.N., Fielding, R.A., Fiatarone, M.A., Meydani, M., Farhengmehr, M., Orencole, S.F., Blumberg, J.B., and Evans, W.J., Acute phase response in exercise, II. Associations between vitamin E, cytokines, and muscle proteolysis, *Am. J. Physiol.*, 260, R1235, 1991.
55. Espersen, G.T., Elbaek, A., Ernst, E., Toft, E., Kaalund, S., Jersild, C., and Grunnet, N., Effect of physical exercise on cytokines and lymphocyte subpopulations in human peripheral blood, *APMIS*, 98, 395, 1990.
56. Bagby, G.J., Sawaya, D.E., Crouch, L.D., and Shepherd, R.E., Prior exercise suppresses the plasma tumor necrosis factor response to bacterial lipopolysaccharide, *J. Appl. Physiol.*, 77(3), 1542, 1994.
57. Drenth, J.P., Van Uum, S.H., Van Deuren, M., Pesman, G.J., Van der Ven-Jongekrijg, J., and Van der Meer, J.W., Endurance run increases circulating IL-6 and IL-1ra but down regulates ex vivo TNF-$\alpha$ and IL-1$\beta$ production, *J. Appl. Physiol.*, 79, 1497, 1995.
58. Sprenger, H., Jacobs, C., Nain, M., Gressner, A.M., Prinz, H., Wesemann, W., and Gemsa, D., Enhanced release of cytokines, interleukin-2 receptors, and neopterin after long-distance running, *Clin. Immunol. Immunopathol.*, 63, 188, 1992.
59. Castell, L.M., Poortmans, J.R., Leclercq, R., Brasseur, M., Duchateau, J., and Newsholme, E.A., Some aspects of the acute phase response after a marathon race, and the effects of glutamine supplementation, *Eur. J. Appl. Physiol.*, 75, 47, 1997.
60. Papanicolaou, D.A., Petrides, J.S., Tsigos, C., Bina, S., Kalogeras, K.T., Wilder, R., Gold, P.W., Deuster, P.A., and Chrousos, G.P., Exercise stimulates interleukin-6 secretion: inhibition by glucocorticoids and correlation with catecholamines, *Am. J. Physiol.*, 271, E601, 1996.
61. Ostrowski, K., Rohde, T., Asp, S., Schjerling, P., and Pedersen, B.K., Pro- and anti-inflammatory cytokine balance in strenuous exercise in humans, *J. Physiol.*, 515, 287, 1999.
62. Ostrowski, K., Hermann, C., Bansash, A., Schjerling, P., Nielsen, J.N., and Pedersen, B.K., A trauma-like elevation of plasma cytokines in humans in response to treadmill running, *J. Physiol.*, 515, 889, 1998.
63. Suzuki, K., Yamada, M., Kurakake, S., Okamura, N., Yamaya, K., Liu, Q., Kudoh, S., Kowatari, K., Nakaji, S., and Sugawara, K., Circulating cytokines and hormones with immunosuppressive but neutrophil-priming potentials rise after endurance exercise in humans, *Eur. J. Appl. Physiol.*, 81, 281, 2000.
64. Camus, G., Nys, M., Poortmans, J.R., Venneman, I., Monfils, T., Deby-Dupont, G., Juchmes-Ferir, A., Deby, C., Lamy, M., and Duchateau, J., Endotoxemia, production of tumor necrosis factor-$\alpha$ and polymorphonuclear neutrophil activation following strenuous exercise in humans, *Eur. J. Appl. Physiol.*, 79, 62, 1998.
65. DeRijk, R., Michelson, M., Karp, B., Petrides, J., Galliven, E., Deuster, P., Paciotti, G., Gold, P.W., and Sternberg, E.M., Exercise and circadian rhythm-induced variations in plasma cortisol differentially regulate interluekin-1$\beta$ (IL-1$\beta$), IL-6, and tumor necrosis factor-$\alpha$ (TNF-$\alpha$) production in humans: high sensitivity of TNF-$\alpha$ and resistance of IL-6, *J. Clin. Endocrinol. Metab.*, 87, 2182, 1997.

66. Coppack, S.W., Pinkey, J.H., and Mohamed-Ali, V., Leptin production in human adipose tissue, *Proc. Nutrition Soc.*, 57, 461, 1998.

67. Zhang, Y, Proenca, R., Maffei, M., Barone, M., Leopold, L., and Friedman, J.M., Positional cloning of the mouse obese gene and its human homologue, *Nature*, 372, 425, 1994.

68. Kennedy, G.C., The role of depot fat in hypothalamic control of food intake in the rat, *Proc. R. Soc.*, 140, 578, 1953.

69. Coleman, D.L., Obese and diabetes: two mutant genes causing diabetes-obesity syndrome in mice, *Diabetologia*, 14, 141, 1978.

70. Caro, J.F., Sinha, M.K., Kolaczynski, J.W., and Zhang, P.L., Leptin: the tale of an obesity gene, *Diabetes*, 45(11),1455, 1996.

71. Pelleymounter, M.A. Cullen, M.J., Baker, M.B., Hecht, R., Winters, D., Boone, T., and Collins, F., Effects of the obese gene product on body weight regulation in ob/ob mice, *Science*, 269, 540, 1995.

72. Halaas, J.L., Gajiwala, K.S., Maffei, M., Cohen, S.L., Chait, B.T., Rabinowitz, D., Lallone, R.L., Burley, S.K., and Friedman, J.M., Weight-reducing effects of the plasma protein encoded by the obese gene, *Science*, 269, 543, 1995.

73. Campfield, L.A., Smith, F.J., Guisez, Y., DeVos, R., and Burn, P., Recombinant mouse OB protein: evidence for a peripheral signal linking adiposity and central neural networks, *Science*, 269, 546, 1995.

74. Wang, J., Liu, R., Hawkins, M., Barzilai, N., and Rosetti, L., A nutrient-sensing pathway regulates leptin gene expression in muscle and fat, *Nature*, 393, 684, 1998.

75. Bado, A., Levasseur, S., Attoub, S., Kermorgant, S., Laigneau, J.P., Borrtoluzzi, M.N., Moizo, L., Lehy, T., Guerre-Millo, M., LeMarchand-Brustel, Y., and Lewin, M.J., The stomach is a source of leptin, *Nature*, 394, 790, 1998.

76. Esler, M., Vaz, M., Collier, G., Nestel, P., Jennings, G., Kaye, D., Seals, D., and Lambert, G., Leptin in human plasma is derived in part from the brain, and cleared by the kidneys, *Lancet*, 351, 879, 1998.

77. Wiesner, G., Vaz, M., Collier, G., Seals, D., Kaye, D., Jennings, G., Lambert, G., Wilkinson, D., and Esler, M., Leptin is released from the human brain: influence of adiposity and gender, *J. Clin. Endocrinol. Metab.*, 84, 2270, 1999.

78. Leclercq, J., Cauzac, M., Lahlou, N., Timsit, J., Girard, J., Auwerx, J., and Haugel de Mouzon, S., Overexpression of placental leptin in diabetic pregnancy: a critical role for insulin, *Diabetes*, 47, 847, 1998.

79. White, D.W. and Tartaglia, L.A., Leptin and OB-R: body weight regulation by a cytokine receptor, *Cytokine Growth Factor Rev.*, 7(9), 303, 1996.

80. Ahima, R.S., Prabakaran, D., Mantzoros, C., Qu, D., Lowell, B.B., Maratos-Flier, E., and Flier, J.S., Role of leptin in the neuroendocrine response to fasting, *Nature*, 382, 250, 1996.

81. Unger, R.H., Zhou, Y., and Orci, L., Regulation of fatty acid homeostasis in cells: novel role of leptin, *Proc. Natl. Acad. Sci. USA*, 96, 2327, 1999.

82. Hickey, M.S., Israel, R.G., Gardiner, S.N., Considine, R.V., McCammon, M.R., Tyndall, G.L., Houmard, J.A., Marks, R.H.L., and Caro, J.F., Gender differences in serum leptin levels in humans, *Biochem. Mol. Med.*, 59, 1, 1996.

83. Tataranni, P.A., Monroe, M.B., Dueck, C.A., Traub, S.A., Nicolson, M., Manore, M.M., Matt, K.S., and Ravussin, E., Adiposity, plasma leptin concentration and reproductive function in active and sedentary females, *Int. J. Obesity Related Metabolic Disorders*, 21(9), 818, 1997.

84. Gippini, A., Mato, A., Peino, R., Lage, M., Dieguez, C., and Casanueva, F.F., Effect of resistance exercise (bodybuilding) training on serum leptin levels in young men. Implications for relationship between body mass index and serum leptin, *J. Endocrinol. Invest.*, 22(11), 824, 1999.

85. Thong, F.S.L., McLean, C., and Graham, T.E., Plasma leptin in female athletes: relationship with body fat, reproductive, nutritional and endocrine factors, *J. Appl. Physiol.*, 88, 2037, 2000.

86. Laughlin, G.A. and Yen, S.S.C., Hypoleptinemia in women athletes: absence of a diurnal rhythm with amenorrhea, *J. Clin. Endocrinol. Metab.*, 82(1), 318, 1997.

87. Hickey, M.S., Considine, R.V., Israel, R.G., Mahar, T.L., McCammon, M.R., Tyndall, G.L., Houmard, J.A., and Caro, J.F., Leptin is related to body fat content in male distance runners, *Am. J. Physiol.*, 271(5, part 1), E938, 1996.

88. Melanson, K.J., Westerterp-Plantenga, M.S., Campfield, L.A., and Saris, W.H., Appetite and blood glucose profiles in humans after glycogen-depleting exercise, *J. Appl. Physiol.*, 87(3), 947, 1999.

89. Perusse, L., Collier, G., Gagnon, J., Leon, A.S., Rao, D.C., Skinner, J.S., Wilmore, J.H., Nadeau, A., Zimmet, P.Z., and Bouchard, C., Acute and chronic effects of exercise on leptin levels in humans, *J. Appl. Physiol.*, 83(1), 5, 1997.

90. Racette, S.B., Coppack, S.W., Landt, M., and Klein, S., Leptin production during moderate-intensity aerobic exercise, *J. Clin. Endocrinol. Metab.*, 82(7), 2275, 1997.

91. Tuominen, J.A., Ebeling, P., Heiman, M.L., Stephens, T., and Koivisto, V.A., Leptin and thermogenesis in humans, *Acta Physiol. Scand.*, 160, 83, 1997.

92. Koistinen, H.A., Tuominen, J.A., Ebeling, P., Heiman, M.L., Stephens, T.W., and Koivisto V.A., The effect of exercise on leptin concentration in healthy men and in type 1 diabetic patients, *Med. Sci. Sports Exerc.*, 30(6), 805, 1998.

93. Kraemer, R.R., Johnson, L.G., Haltom, R., Kraemer, G.R., Hebert, E.P., Gimpel, T., and Castracane, V.D., Serum leptin concentrations in response to acute exercise in postmenopausal women with and without hormone replacement therapy, *Proc. Soc. Exper. Biol. Med.*, 221(3), 171, 1999.

94. Landt, M., Lawson, G.M., Helgeson, J.M., Davila-Roman, V.G., Ladenson, J.H., Jaffe, A.S., and Hickner, R.C., Prolonged exercise decreases serum leptin concentration, *Metab. Clin. Exper.*. 46(10), 1109, 1997.

95. Leal-Cerro, A., Garcia-Luna, P.P., Astorga, R., Parejo, J., Peino, R., Dieguez, C., and Casanueva, F.F., Serum leptin levels in male marathon athletes before and after the marathon run, *J. Clin. Endocrinol. Metab.*, 83(7), 2376, 1998.

96. Tuominen, J.A., Ebeling, P., Laquier, F.W., Heiman, M.L., Stephens, T., and Koivisto V.A., Serum leptin concentration and fuel homeostasis in healthy man, *Eur. J. Clin. Invest.*, 27(3), 206, 1997.

97. Dirlewanger, M., Di Vetta, V., Giusti, V., Schneiter, P., Jequier, E., and Tappy, L., Effect of moderate physical activity on plasma leptin concentration in humans, *Eur. J. Appl. Physiol. Occup. Physiol.*, 79(4), 331, 1999.

98. Ryan, A.S., Pratley, R.E., Elahi, D., and Goldberg, A.P., Changes in plasma leptin and insulin action with resistive training in postmenopausal women, *Int. J. Obesity Related Metab. Disorders*, 24(1), 27, 2000.

99. Kohrt, W.M., Landt, M., Birge, Jr., S.J., Serum leptin levels are reduced in response to exercise training, but not hormone replacement therapy, in older women, *J. Clin. Endocrinol. Metab.*, 81(11), 3980, 1996.

100. Kraemer, R.R., Kraemer, G.R., Acevedo, E.O., Hebert, E.P., Temple, E., Bates, M., Etie, A., Haltom, R., Quinn, S., and Castracane, V.D., Effects of aerobic exercise on serum leptin levels in obese women, *Eur. J. Appl. Physiol. Occup. Physiol.*, 80(2), 154, 1999.

101. Okazaki, T., Himeno, E., Nanri, H., Ogata, H., and Ikeda, M., Effects of mild aerobic exercise and a mild hypocaloric diet on plasma leptin in sedentary women, *Clin. Exp. Pharmacol. Physiol.*, 26(5-6), 415, 1999.

102. Hickey, M.S., Houmard, J.A., Considine, R.V., Tyndall, G.L., Midgette, J.B., Gavigan, K.E., Weidner, M.L., McCammon, M.R., Israel, R.G., and Caro, J.F. Gender-dependent effects of exercise training on serum leptin levels in humans, *Am. J. Physiol.*, 272(4, part 1), E562, 1997.

103. Pasman, W.J., Westerterp-Plantenga, M.S., and Saris, W.H., The effect of exercise training on leptin levels in obese males, *Am. J. Physiol.*, 274(2, part 1), E280, 1998.

104. van Aggel-Leijssen, D.P., van Baak, M.A., Tenenbaum, R., Campfield, L.A., and Saris, W.H., Regulation of average 24-hr human plasma leptin level: the influence of exercise and physiological changes in energy balance, *Int. J. Obesity Related Metabolic Disorders*, 23(2), 151, 1999.

105. Hilton, L.K. and Loucks, A.B., Low energy availability, not exercise stress, suppresses the diurnal rhythm of leptin in healthy young women, *Am. J. Physiol. Endocrinol. Metab.*, 278(1), E43, 2000.

106. Mueller, W.M., Gregoire, F.M., Stanhope, K.L., Mobbs, C.V., Mizuno, T.M., Warden, C.H., Stern, J.S., and Havel, P.J., Evidence that glucose metabolism regulates leptin secretion from cultured adipocytes, *Endocrinology*, 139, 551, 1998.

107. Sarraf, P., Frederich, R.C., Turner, E.M., Ma, G., Jaskowiak, N.T., Rivet, 3rd., D.J. Flier, J.S., Lowell, B.B., Fraker, D.L., and Alexander, H.R., Multiple cytokines and acute inflammation raise mouse leptin levels: potential role in inflammatory anorexia, *J. Exp. Med.*, 185(1), 171, 1997.

108. Grunfeld, C., Zhao, C., Fuller, J., Pollack, A., Moser, A., Friedman, J., and Feingold, K.R., Endotoxin and cytokines induce expression of leptin, the *ob* gene product, in hamsters, *J. Clin. Invest.*, 97, 2152, 1996.

109. Chin-Chance, C., Polonsky, K.S., and Schoeller, D.A., Twenty-four-hour leptin levels respond to cumulative short-term energy imbalance and predict subsequent intake, *J. Clin. Endocrinol. Metab.*, 85, 2685, 2000.

110. Brabant, G., Horn, R., von zur Muhlen, A., Mayr, B., Wurster, U., Heidenreich, F., Schnabel, D., Gruters-Kieslich, A., Zimmermann-Belsing, T., and Feldt-Rasmussen, U., Free- and protein-bound leptin are distinct and independently controlled factors in energy regulation, *Diabetologia*, 43, 438, 2000.

*chapter six*

# Effects of endurance exercise on total body adiposity in adults

*Alice S. Ryan*

## Contents

0-8493-0460-1/02/$0.00+$1.50
© 2002 by CRC Press LLC

## 6.1   Introduction

A sedentary lifestyle results in numerous physiologic and functional declines that increase risk for disease. Obesity and weight gain in sedentary adults are strongly associated with the development of hypertension, hyperlipidemia, and insulin resistance, which are risk factors for cardiovascular disease (CVD). Adults should sustain physical activity to perhaps prevent the age-associated increases in weight gain and fat mass. Aerobic exercise training provides numerous health benefits to adults, including increases in physical fitness and well-being, reductions in blood pressure, improvements in lipoprotein lipid profiles and glucose metabolism, and increases in bone mineral density. The focus of this chapter is to provide a review of the studies that have examined the effects of aerobic or endurance exercise training on adiposity, specifically total body fat, in order to better understand if beneficial body composition changes result from aerobic exercise training.

## 6.2   Body composition

### 6.2.1   Health impact of obesity

Currently, 66% of men and 55% of women in the U.S. are considered overweight or obese as defined by a body mass index (BMI) $\geq 25$ kg/m.[1,2] Moreover, the prevalence of obesity (BMI $\geq 30$ kg/m$^2$) continues to increase in the U.S., with an approximate 6% increase from 1991 to 1998; the greatest magnitude of increase is found among 18 to 29 year olds, those with some college education, and those of Hispanic ethnicity.[2] The significant changes in body weight and composition that occur from adulthood to older age affect health and can increase the propensity for disease. Specifically, the increase in obesity is associated with increased prevalence of cardiovascular disease, hypertension, gallbladder disease, osteoarthritis, and type 2 diabetes.[2]

Severe obesity is associated with increased mortality.[3] In other studies, the association between body weight and mortality is either not apparent[4] or shows a J-shaped curve,[5] a U-shaped relationship,[6] or a direct association.[7,8] In women, the lowest mortality was observed among lean women after accounting for cigarette smoking and disease-related weight loss.[9] In addition, weight gain of 10 kg or more after the age of 18 is associated with increased mortality in middle adulthood.[9] Although these studies focus on body weight or use BMI as a measure of obesity, a direct association between fat mass and all-cause and CVD death rates in men was recently reported.[10] Not only is obesity related to increased mortality, but also a low level of physical fitness is associated with increased risk of all-cause and CVD mortality.[11-14] Men who improve their physical fitness reduce their mortality risk by ~44%.[15] Furthermore, both beginning a moderately vigorous sports activity and avoiding obesity are separately associated with lower death rates from all causes and from CVD in middle-aged and older men.[5] All-cause mortality risk is also reduced by physical activity in postmenopausal women.[16] Middle-aged women who maintained a healthy lifestyle (e.g., not overweight, exercised moderately or vigorously 30 min/day, did not smoke, ate a healthy diet, and consumed alcohol moderately) had a greater than 80% reduction in the incidence of coronary events compared to the remainder of women in the population studied.[17] Moreover, brisk walking and vigorous exercise are associated with considerable and similar risk reductions in the incidence of coronary events among women,[18] suggesting that performance of regular moderate-intensity exercise that is realistic, safe, and attainable for most individuals provides enormous health benefits.

## 6.2.2   Effects of aging

Body weight is composed of the sum of a variety of tissues, the largest component being body water, which comprises approximately 60% of body weight. Body water can be further divided into intracellular (40%) and extracellular (20%) components. The remaining cellular components of the body are lipids, proteins, glycogen, and minerals. At the tissue level, these body components are adipose tissue, skeletal muscle, visceral organs, and bone. In healthy people, body weight and fat mass increase gradually from early adulthood until the fifth to sixth decade, after which weight tends to plateau. The Gerontology Research Center of the National Institute of Aging developed age-specific, weight-for-height ranges that are applicable to men and women and are recommended by the National Research Council and the U.S. Department of Agriculture. The table[19] allows for increases in weight by decade (approximately 4 kg) from 20 to 69 years. Body weight increased 2.1 kg per decade in a cross-sectional sample of almost 1500 men ages 25 to 70 years.[20] Similarly, in a cross-sectional analysis of women ages 20 to 64 years, an increase in body weight of 2.8 kg per decade was entirely due to an increase in body fat.[20] However, the increases in body weight and body fat were slightly less (+1.8 kg) in women who were longitudinally followed for ~3.5 years.[20] In the Fels Longitudinal Study, the age-related increase in body weight was ~0.3 kg/yr in men and ~0.55 kg/yr in women, with increases in total body fat of ~0.37 kg/yr and ~0.41 kg/yr, respectively.[21] Hence, increases in body weight and body fat can occur with aging. The objective would be to prevent, slow, or modify these changes in body composition in adults, perhaps by endurance exercise training.

## 6.2.3   Measurement of body fat

Body composition may be assessed by a variety of methods including anthropometry (circumferences, skinfolds), hydrodensitometry, bioelectrical impedance (BIA), dual-energy X-ray absorptiometry (DXA), computed tomography, magnetic resonance imaging, *in vivo* neutron activation analysis, determining total body potassium, and the isotope dilution method (total body water). Combinations of these methodologies to estimate the different components of the body lend way to three- and four-compartment models of body composition assessment;[22] however, a discussion of these method-ologies is beyond the scope of this chapter. The reader is referred to excellent reviews[19,22–24] for complete descriptions of the use, methods, assumptions, limitations, and strengths of these methodologies. In this chapter, the par-ticular body composition emphasis is on the change in total body fat. In general, studies of this nature have determined adiposity by hydrodensito-metry, DXA, BIA, and the sum of skinfolds. Hydrodensitometry and DXA have been compared and validated for the measurement of fat mass in young adults,[25] young and older subjects,[26] and elderly adults (>70 years).[27] Fur-thermore, comparisons of DXA with BMI and BIA for estimating fat mass have also been made in men across the age span.[28] DXA can also provide an accurate estimate of whole-body composition in obese subjects (BMI ~ 45 kg/m²) using half-body scans.[29] Yet, caution is warranted regarding the use of anthropometric estimation methods in research settings due to the high individual variability associated with these methods in adults.[26] Most of these methodologies, however, can be reasonably and accurately employed to assess differences in adiposity between individuals who regu-larly exercise vs. those who do not, and to determine changes in body fat with endurance exercise training in adults.

## 6.3   Aerobic exercise and total body fat

### 6.3.1   Cross-sectional studies

#### 6.3.1.1   Athletes vs. sedentary individuals

Reports of studies to determine differences between endurance-trained ath-letes or physically fit individuals vs. sedentary adults provide some insight into the effects of endurance exercise training on adiposity. Sedentary young men and premenopausal women have higher body fat levels than men and women of similar age who regularly perform endurance exercise.[30–35] In addition, when young collegiate athletes of low body weight relative to height (BMI < 20.3 kg/m²) were matched by age, height, and weight to sedentary adults, the athletes had ~5 kg less body fat mass and almost a 10% lower percent body fat by hydrodensitometry than the low-body-weight sedentary adults.[36] These differences were magnified when the ath-letes were compared to normal-weight sedentary adults; the sedentary indi-viduals had more than twice the fat mass and ~13% greater percent body fat.[36] In our study of female athletes (swimmers, runners, triathletes), per-cent body fat was 9% greater and fat mass was ~4 kg higher by DXA in sedentary young women than young athletes, even though the BMIs were remarkably similar.[33] Young, sedentary males have higher body fat than male long-distance runners.[32] Even athletes of various sports may have different body fat levels. Male water polo players have higher fat mass than judo and karate athletes.[30]

Greater adiposity is also observed in older sedentary individuals than older athletes.[33–35,37–41] Male older athletes who had trained on average for more than 20 years had ~5% lower body fat and 5 kg lower body fat mass than lean (body fat < 25%) sedentary males.[37] This difference was exaggerated to reflect a twofold difference in percent fat and a 15-kg difference in fat mass between the athletes and obese sedentary men.[37] Although lean untrained males were ~13% below average weight for their age and height, they had a greater (~4.5%) fat content than master athletes.[40] These studies[37,40] suggest that even when sedentary men are recruited to be "lean," they have higher body fat than athletes, and adiposity differences are inflated between athletes and untrained average men and women. Body fat is also higher in unfit men than fit men in a large cohort of lean, normal, and obese men ages 30 to 83 years.[10] Other studies demonstrating greater body fat in older sedentary men than male athletes indicate that these differences in percent body fat range between ~6 and 10%.[38,39] Sedentary postmenopausal women have higher levels of body fat mass by skinfolds[35] and DXA[33,34,41] than older endurance-trained women. In fact, athletic postmenopausal women had a relative 33% lower body fat and 36% lower fat mass than older sedentary women.[41] Absolute percent body fat is ~12 to 14% higher in older sedentary women of various age groups than endurance-trained women.[33,35] Men and women who were physically active had significantly lower total body fat than men and women who had low physical activity levels.[21] Thus, comparisons within age groups and gender indicate that both young and older sedentary men and women have greater total body adiposity than young and older athletic or physically active men and women, respectively.

### 6.3.1.2    Young vs. older athletes

Because differences in body fat exist between athletes and sedentary individuals of similar age, it is possible that maintenance of an active lifestyle would prevent the increase in adiposity with age such that older, highly trained athletes still benefit from their continued endurance exercise training. In young and middle-aged adult female distance runners, no age-associated differences in total body fat have been observed.[42,43] In highly trained women athletes, no differences in percent fat and total fat mass by DXA were found between the younger (~20 years) and older (~58 years) women athletes.[33] Similarly, the mean estimated body fat by skinfolds was virtually identical between young (~26 years) and master (~60 years) male athletes.[38] In another study,[44] percent body fat did not differ in male master runners across 10-year age groups from 40 to >70 years but was greater in women athletes who were 60+ years old than in 40-year-old women athletes.

In contrast, other studies report an increase in adiposity with age in active adults. An increase in total body adiposity with age has been described in active women.[34,45] Yet, these increases in total body fat in women who regularly perform endurance exercise are modest and are smaller than the increase observed in healthy, sedentary women.[34] It has been suggested that declines in energy expenditure with aging may explain these results,[45] but a reduction in exercise volume did not explain the age-associated increase in total body fat in active women.[34] In other studies, male master runners had higher body fat than elite young runners.[40,46-48] Proctor and Joyner[49] reported an age-associated increase in percent body fat between young (~25 years) and older (~64 years) chronically endurance-trained men and women. In another study,[50] the level of physical activity (0 to ~1500 kcal/day) did not predict percent body fat by BIA in healthy elderly men and women. The authors[50] suggest that a more intensive exercise regimen than what is performed by many elderly individuals may be necessary to decrease body fat without a change in diet. This may explain why older men and women athletes who train vigorously more than 5 days/week have very low percent body fat (~11 and 23%, respectively).[33,38] Even though some of these studies suggest that older athletes may have higher body fat levels than young athletes, it should be noted that older endurance athletes have lower body fat than is average for young individuals.[51]

### 6.3.1.3   Summary
The majority of studies suggest that physically active adults have lower levels of body fat than sedentary individuals and that maintenance or current high levels of physical fitness may reduce increases in adiposity that may normally occur during adulthood. Because of the inherent biases of cross-sectional studies, prospective studies are needed to fully and clearly elucidate whether body fat is reduced by an increase in endurance physical activity.

## 6.3.2   Longitudinal studies

### 6.3.2.1   Follow-up of athletes
Several studies have followed athletes for many years to observe whether changes in adiposity, as determined by skinfold measurements, occur as the athletes age.[51-55] Percent fat did not change over an 8-year period in male master athletes.[55] In contrast, a 10-year follow-up of male master athletes (50 to 82 years) showed a significant but small (+2%) increase in percent body fat regardless of whether the men remained competitive or had become noncompetitive and reduced their training intensities.[51] Two other longitudinal follow-up studies demonstrated that whole body adiposity increased with age in elite athletic men even though they maintained high levels of endurance exercise.[52,53] Specifically, percent body fat increased approximately 2 to 3% per decade in older men who remained active over the 20- to 22-year period.[52,53] A 15-year follow-up of elite male athletes showed that those runners who maintained a current running program had not changed body fat, whereas those former athletes who had stopped training had significantly increased body fat.[54] Moreover, body fat of the former athletes was not different than sedentary controls, suggesting that a decline in physical training influences a gain in body fat to levels similar to individuals who had never been athletes. This was confirmed by Pollock and colleagues,[53] who concluded that changes in body composition were related to a reduction in training habits, but, importantly, these increases in percent body fat were

less than those observed in a healthy sedentary population. All of the above studies were conducted in men. Reports of longitudinal follow-up of female athletes are lacking.

### 6.3.2.2   Endurance exercise training

Over the past 50 years, numerous studies have examined changes in total body adiposity with endurance exercise training. In several studies, endurance exercise training can result in losses in body fat with minimal or no changes in body weight.[56–60] Young, sedentary, non-obese men lost weight, had a decrease in the sum of skinfolds, and lost 2.6 kg of fat mass and percent body fat after 20 weeks of intense aerobic training.[60] Men ages 17 to 59 years who jogged 3 days/week for 10 weeks had small decreases in body weight (–1 kg) and percent body fat (–1%) by hydrodensitometry.[56] Healthy 70- to 79-year-old men and women lost minimal body weight (1 kg) but had a significant decrease in the sum of seven skinfolds and estimated percent body fat (~–4%) after 6 months of endurance exercise training 3 times a week at 75 to 85% heart rate reserve.[57] Similarly, middle-aged women who completed a 12-week "brisk" walking program (20 to 50 min, 2 to 3 times a week) lost only 1 kg body mass but had a decrease in the sum of four skinfolds.[58] In a study of male and female diabetics, endurance exercise training (30 to 45 min, 3 to 4 times a week) resulted in a significant 2.3% decrease in percent body fat at 3 months and an additional 1.1% decrease at the end of 6 months of training with no changes in body weight.[59]

Certain subject characteristics and aspects of the training program may influence whether changes in total body adiposity occur after individuals undergo an endurance exercise regime. These include the age, baseline adiposity, gender, and genetics of the participants as well as the duration of the training program, the energy expenditure of the exercise, and the type of exercise program. These factors and how they affect body composition changes are described in the following sections.

### 6.3.2.2.1   Age of subjects.

The question arises as to whether differences in study population (e.g., young vs. old) could affect whether losses in adiposity occur with endurance exercise training. In young, healthy, mildly overweight men, 6 months of endurance exercise training (45 min at 85% heart rate reserve, 5 times a week) did not change body weight or total body fat mass.[61] However, the same intensive program significantly decreased body weight by 2.5 kg, percent body fat by 2.3%, and fat mass by 2.4 kg in older overweight men.[61] This would suggest that there might be an age effect of the response to endurance exercise training. Conversely, premenopausal obese women who performed aerobic exercise 4 to 5 times a week for 14 months at ~55% $VO_2max$, lost on average 4.6 kg of body fat as measured by hydrodensitometry.[62] This loss was even less than expected due to the cost of the energy expenditure of the exercise training program. In two studies involving elderly subjects (~60 to 80 years), the loss of body weight averaged approximately 2 to 2.5 kg, with an approximate 1% drop

in percent body fat and an 11% decrease in fat mass after 6 months[63] and
9 months[64] of training. Moreover, in a review of studies involving aerobic
training in older individuals, aerobic exercise decreased fat mass between
–0.4 and –3.2 kg in 20 of the 22 studies reviewed.[65] Thus, losses of body fat
have been reported in young and older individuals after endurance exercise
training. Age does not appear to be a significant factor for changes in adiposity with endurance exercise training.

   6.3.2.2.2   *Baseline adiposity of subjects.*   Could baseline body fat levels
predict whether changes in body fat occur as a result of endurance exercise
training? Several studies would suggest that this may be true. Changes in
the sum of skinfold thickness after 6 weeks of intensive military training
were related to the initial skinfold thickness in thin, normal, and obese male
army recruits.[66] Although a 5-day/week, moderate-intensity, intermittent
walking program for 32 weeks was not sufficient to induce a loss of body
weight or body fat in overweight and obese women older than approximately 43 years, those women who had the greatest body fat at baseline lost
body fat, albeit a relatively small amount (<1 kg).[67] Moreover, young type 1
diabetic men, who were not obese, did not lose body fat estimated by the
sum of skinfolds after participating in a 12- to 16-week aerobic training
program.[68] Similarly, middle-aged, type 2 diabetic men, also not obese, had
no significant changes in body weight, fat mass, or percent fat by hydrodensitometry after 3 and 6 months of aerobic training.[69] In a small sample
of normal weight-for-height elderly men and women, 16 weeks of cycling
training did not change body weight but had a tendency to result in a loss
of body fat ($p = 0.07$).[70] Neither body weight nor body fat was altered in
elderly (60 to 80 years), healthy, normal to overweight (BMI average of
~25 kg/m$^2$) men and women who underwent 6 months of aerobic training
3 to 4 times a week.[70]
   Obese individuals, on the other hand, have benefited with respect to
changes in adiposity after participating in endurance exercise training programs.[61,62,71–74] A 9- to 12-month endurance training program resulted in a
significant loss of body weight, percent fat, and fat mass (~3 and 1.5 kg) in
overweight older men and women, respectively.[74] These losses were less than
expected from the energy cost of the exercise, partially due to an increase in
caloric intake.[74] Young, obese men lost almost 6 kg body fat by hydrodensitometry after a 16-week vigorous walking program.[71] Furthermore, obese
male military recruits had an ~12-kg loss of fat mass after a 20-week basic
training program.[75] Obese women have also lost body fat after aerobic exercise programs of 17 weeks[72] and 1 year.[73] In two studies[76,77] involving obese
men, the reduction in total fat was greater in an exercise weight-loss group
than a group that underwent dietary intervention. Furthermore, the losses
in body fat were large and averaged 6 to 8 kg over a 12-week period. Very
large decreases in fat mass (~11 kg) have also been reported in obese women
after only 45 days of endurance exercise training.[78] A meta-analysis, which
included 40 studies where body fat changes were measured in obese adults

after approximately 20 weeks of endurance exercise training, indicated that an average loss of 3 kg of body fat occurred with the exercise programs.[79]

Others contend that exercise training may not result in weight loss in obese subjects or, if exercise training does reduce body mass and fat mass, the changes are relatively small.[80] In one study, overweight and obese postmenopausal women who walked for 12 weeks (1 hour/day, 5 times a week) failed to lose body weight or body fat by DXA.[81] Yet, the same training program resulted in a significant 1.5-kg decrease in body weight and 1.3-kg decrease in fat mass in similarly obese, postmenopausal women but who had type 2 diabetes. This difference could not be explained, and it was not due to compliance or to the increases in $VO_2$max, which were similar between normoglycemic and diabetic women. Moreover, obese women failed to lose body weight or change body composition after a 12-week, low-intensity exercise training program.[82] In a more robust manner than examining studies individually, Ballor and Keesey[83] performed a meta-analysis of 53 aerobic exercise training studies published between 1950 and 1988. They showed that, for both males and females, initial body fat levels accounted for a large portion of the variance associated with changes in weight, fat mass, and percent fat. In their analyses, the reduction in fat mass averaged –1.5 kg with a –1.7% reduction in percent body fat.[83] Thus, these studies would suggest that normal-weight individuals may either not lose body fat with endurance exercise or, if they do, these changes may be negligible and that individuals with the greatest adiposity may lose more body fat with endurance exercise training.

*6.3.2.2.3 Gender of subjects.* Reductions in fat mass with exercise training may also be gender dependent. Animal studies first reported that losses of body weight are greater in male rats than female rats. Female rats tend to preserve body mass by increasing energy intake during exercise, whereas exercised male rats decrease food intake,[84-86] suggesting that the females were more resistant to the exercise program. However, exercise did decrease percent body fat in both male and female rats.[85] In a meta-analysis of over 50 studies, males lost more body weight than females for running/walking exercise, but this disparity might be partially due to the fact that the energy expenditure per session was reportedly twice as high in the men than women.[83] Unfortunately, losses in body fat, specifically comparing men and women, were not examined in this report. In other recent studies, the loss of fat mass was smaller in women than men.[87-91,92] After men and women participated in an exercise program for 50 min/day, 3 times a week for 3 months, the men had decreased their body fat, but body fat tended to increase in women.[89] Moreover, Westerterp and co-workers[93] showed that the loss of fat mass was significantly less in women than men as the women tended to preserve their energy balance during a 40-week training for a half-marathon. In the HERITAGE family study, fat loss was significantly greater in men compared with women (–0.9 vs. –0.5 kg) after 20 weeks of aerobic training.[91] It is clear that additional research is necessary to delineate whether the effects of endurance exercise training on total body adiposity vary by gender.

   *6.3.2.2.4  Genetic background of subjects.*  The magnitude of the effect of exercise training on body fat may be attributed to heredity.[88,94] In an innovative experiment, Bouchard et al.[94] studied young adult male twins over 93 days, during which the men performed cycle exercise 9 out of every 10 days and nutrient intake was kept constant. The 5-kg weight loss was synergistic with a 4.9-kg loss of fat mass and a 4.8% drop in percent body fat. Interestingly, the changes in adiposity were more similar within twin pairs than between twin pairs, suggesting that loss of body fat with aerobic exercise training may be affected by genotype. In the HERITAGE family study, 20 weeks of cycle ergometer exercise training resulted in small, but statistically significant, changes in total adiposity as measured by anthropometry.[95] The putative gene for these changes in fat mass was dominant and accounted for 31% of the variance in the change in adiposity.[96] The transmissibility estimates for the response phenotypes ranged between 15 and 20%, and the response among subjects of the same generation were more similar than in subjects of different generations. The authors suggest that this could occur from familial genetic and/or environmental factors that are age dependent.[95]

   In summary, certain subject characteristics can alter changes in body composition with endurance exercise training. Nevertheless, the loss of body fat in overweight and obese adults may also be dependent on aspects of the training regime including the duration and energy expenditure of the exercise program.[83] Thus, facets of the exercise program may also be critical to the success of aerobic training programs to induce total body adiposity losses.

   *6.3.2.2.5  Duration of training program.*  Numerous studies[76,77,97–102] have compared diet and exercise interventions on losses in body weight and fat mass. In general, it is apparent from these studies that changes in body fat do occur with aerobic training, but vary from 1 to 8 kg and may be dependent on the length of the training program. For example, after 10 weeks of exercise, normal-weight men had a 1-kg loss in body fat,[98] whereas obese men, who exercised for 3 months, lost approximately 3.5 kg of fat mass.[100] Sedentary, young women randomized to a 3 to 4 times a week aerobic training program for 13 weeks had a significant loss of percent body fat (–4%) and fat mass (–2.5 kg).[102] Sedentary, overweight, middle-aged men and women who participated in a 3 to 4 times a week, 6-month aerobic training program at 70 to 85% heart rate reserve lost ~1.8 kg body weight and showed a 1.6% drop in percent body fat.[97] These losses contrasted the lack of change in a control group. Aerobic training studies of longer duration (~1 year) resulted in slightly greater losses in fat mass (4 kg) in overweight men.[99,101] A meta-analysis examining the exercise-induced changes in body fat specified that the duration of the exercise (minutes/session) and weeks of training were significant predictors of change in percent fat in females.[83] This was confirmed in a recent review of aerobic training studies in older adults, which indicated that losses of fat mass were related to the duration of the exercise program (e.g., total number of sessions).[65] Therefore, the amount of exercise performed is an important determinant of the changes in body composition with aerobic training and requires consideration when comparing endurance exercise training studies and changes in fat mass.

*6.3.2.2.6 Energy expenditure of the exercise.* It is conceivable that differences in exercise intensity may play a role in the loss of body fat with aerobic exercise training. Tremblay et al.[90] compared the effects of a 20-week continuous cycling program (~45 min) and a 15-week, high-intensity, intermittent endurance exercise training program in young men and women on subcutaneous fat as determined by the sum of six skinfolds. Neither program resulted in a loss of body weight. Only the intermittent, high-intensity exercise program elicited a significant loss of body fat. This occurred despite the fact that the total energy expenditure of the continuous cycling protocol was twice that of the interval cycling protocol. These results suggest that fat loss is greater when exercise intensity is high. In contrast, when older, sedentary men and women were randomized to either high-intensity (40 min at 73 to 88% peak heart rate) or low-intensity (30 min at 60 to 73% peak heart rate), home-based treadmill exercise for 3 times a week, no significant changes in body weight or fat occurred in either group.[103] Nonetheless, in a meta-analysis of over 50 studies, exercise energy expenditure accounted for more than 50% of the variance in exercise-induced changes in fat mass and percent fat.[83]

*6.3.2.2.7 Type of exercise program.* Variations in the exercise protocol and the setting where the training takes place may also impact the loss of body fat with endurance exercise training. Donnelly et al.[104] compared the effects of 18 months of continuous (30 min of exercise, 3 times a week, at 60 to 75% $VO_2$max) vs. intermittent (two 15-min brisk walking sessions, 5 times a week) exercise on body composition in moderately obese females. Only those women who underwent the continuous exercise protocol had a significant decrease in percent body fat (~2%) and fat mass (–2 kg). In a randomized trial comparing three treadmill exercise protocols (long-bout exercise, multiple short-bout exercise, or multiple short-bout exercise with home exercise equipment) in sedentary, overweight young women, significant losses in body weight and body fat occurred in all groups after 18 months of training.[105] Participants lost ~6 kg of body fat by 6 months, with the greatest change in percent body fat and fat mass being found in the short-bout exercise with home equipment group. These results suggest that having access to home exercise equipment may improve compliance and is more effective in weight loss and fat loss in adult women. In another recent trial,[106] sedentary men and women were randomized to either a structured exercise program or a lifestyle program. The structured program consisted of supervised sessions at 50 to 80% maximal aerobic power for 20 to 60 min. In the lifestyle program, participants were encouraged to accumulate >30 min of moderate-intensity exercise and attended classes on cognitive and behavioral strategies related to physical activity behavior. A significant loss of percent body fat at 6 months was observed with both programs. The same participants maintained these different exercise programs for an additional 18 months.[107] Percent body fat decreased significantly from baseline in both intervention groups after 24 months of exercise.[107] However, percent body fat decreased (−1.13%) from 6 to 24 months in the lifestyle group and did not change in the structured exercise group (−0.07%). Yet, importantly, the participants did not gain weight during a maintenance period when many individuals would tend to gain weight. Thus, differences in the type of exercise program may contribute to whether individuals lose body fat and maintain these losses.

## 6.4   Summary and recommendations

The American College of Sports Medicine (ACSM) and Centers for Disease Control[108] recommend that adults engage in 30 minutes or more of moderate physical activity most, if not all, days of the week. Such an exercise prescription will result in important health benefits. This chapter examined the effects of endurance exercise training on total body adiposity. In general, cross-sectional studies conclude that sedentary individuals have greater adiposity than individuals who exercise regularly or who are competitive athletes. Longitudinal studies demonstrate that numerous factors may contribute to whether losses in total body adiposity occur as a result of endurance exercise training. These include, but are not limited to, the subject characteristics (gender, baseline adiposity, genetic background) and aspects of the exercise program (duration, intensity, and the type of exercise). The majority of studies reflect that exercise training has the potential to alter body composition, although it may be a relatively modest loss of body fat. Nevertheless, minimal changes in body fat could positively impact the prevention and treatment of disease, especially those strongly associated with obesity, such as diabetes, hypertension, and hyperlipidemia. Thus, physical activity should become and/or remain an integral part of every adult's lifestyle.

## Acknowledgments

This research was supported by funds from NIH grant K01-AG00747 and the Department of Veterans Affairs, Baltimore Geriatric Research, Education and Clinical Center (GRECC), Baltimore, Maryland.

# *References*

1. Must, A., Spadano, J., Coakley, E.H., Field, A.E., Colditz, G., and Dietz, W.H., The disease burden associated with overweight and obesity, *JAMA*, 282, 1523, 1999.
2. Mokdad, A.H., Serdula, M.K., Dietz, W.H., Bowman, B.A., Marks, J.S., and Koplan, J.P., The spread of the obesity epidemic in the United States, 1991–1998, *JAMA*, 282, 1519, 1999.
3. Van Itallie, T.B., Obesity: adverse effects on health and longevity, *Am. J. Clin. Nutr.*, 32, 2723, 1979.
4. Vandenbroucke, J.P., Mauritz, B.J., de Bruin, A., Verheesen, J.H., Heide-Wessel, C., and van der Heide, R.M., Weight, smoking, and mortality, *JAMA*, 252, 2859, 1984.
5. Paffenbarger, Jr., R.S., Hyde, R.T., Wing, A.L., Lee, I.M., Jung, D.L., and Kampert, J.B., The association of changes in physical activity level and other lifestyle characteristics with mortality among men, *N. Engl. J. Med.*, 328, 538, 1993.
6. Harris, T., Cook, E.F., Garrison, R., Higgins, M., Kannel, W., and Goldman, L., Body mass index and mortality among nonsmoking older persons. The Framingham Heart Study, *JAMA*, 259, 1520, 1988.
7. Lindsted, K., Tonstad, S., and Kuzma, J.W., Body mass index and patterns of mortality among Seventh-Day Adventist men, *Int. J. Obesity*, 15, 397, 1991.
8. Lee, I.M., Manson, J.E., Hennekens, C.H., and Paffenbarger, Jr., R.S., Body weight and mortality. A 27-year follow-up of middle-aged men, *JAMA*, 270, 2823, 1993.
9. Manson, J.E., Willett, W.C., Stampfer, M.J., Colditz, G.A., Hunter, D.J., Hankinson, S.E., Hennekens, C.H., and Speizer, F.E., Body weight and mortality among women, *N. Engl. J. Med.*, 333, 677, 1995.
10. Lee, C.D., Blair, S.N., and Jackson, A.S., Cardiorespiratory fitness, body composition, and all-cause and cardiovascular disease mortality in men, *Am. J. Clin. Nutr.*, 69, 373, 1999.
11. Ekelund, L.G., Haskell, W.L., Johnson, J.L., Whaley, F.S., Criqui, M.H., and Sheps, D.S., Physical fitness as a predictor of cardiovascular mortality in asymptomatic North American men. The Lipid Research Clinics Mortality Follow-up Study, *N. Engl. J. Med.*, 319, 1379, 1988.
12. Lie, H., Mundal, R., and Erikssen, J., Coronary risk factors and incidence of coronary death in relation to physical fitness. Seven-year follow-up study of middle-aged and elderly men, *Eur. Heart J.*, 6, 147, 1985.
13. Sandvik, L., Erikssen, J., Thaulow, E., Erikssen, G., Mundal, R., and Rodahl, K., Physical fitness as a predictor of mortality among healthy, middle-aged Norwegian men, *N. Engl. J. Med.*, 328, 533, 1993.
14. Wei, M., Kampert, J.B., Barlow, C.E., Nichaman, M.Z., Gibbons, L.W., Paffenbarger, Jr., R.S., and Blair, S.N., Relationship between low cardiorespiratory fitness and mortality in normal-weight, overweight, and obese men, *JAMA*, 282, 1547, 1999.
15. Blair, S.N., Kohl, III, H.W., Barlow, C.E., Paffenbarger, Jr., R.S., Gibbons, L.W., and Macera, C.A., Changes in physical fitness and all-cause mortality. A prospective study of healthy and unhealthy men, *JAMA*, 273, 1093, 1995.

16. Kushi, L.H., Fee, R.M., Folsom, A.R., Mink, P.J., Anderson, K.E., and Sellers, T.A., Physical activity and mortality in postmenopausal women, *JAMA*, 277, 1287, 1997.

17. Stampfer, M.J., Hu, F.B., Manson, J.E., Rimm, E.B., and Willett, W.C., Primary prevention of coronary heart disease in women through diet and lifestyle, *N. Engl. J. Med.*, 343, 16, 2000.

18. Manson, J.E., Hu, F.B., Rich-Edwards, J.W., Colditz, G.A., Stampfer, M.J., Willett, W.C., Speizer, F.E., and Hennekens, C.H., A prospective study of walking as compared with vigorous exercise in the prevention of coronary heart disease in women, *N. Engl. J. Med.*, 341, 650, 1999.

19. Ryan, A.S. and Elahi, D., *Body: Composition, Weight, Height, and Build*, Academic Press, Inc., San Diego, CA, 1996, p. 193.

20. Jackson, A.S., Beard, E.F., Wier, L.T., Ross, R.M., Stuteville, J.E., and Blair, S.N., Changes in aerobic power of men, ages 25–70 yr, *Med. Sci. Sports Exerc.*, 27, 113, 1995.

21. Guo, S.S., Zeller, C., Chumlea, W.C., and Siervogel, R.M., Aging, body composition, and lifestyle: the Fels Longitudinal Study, *Am. J. Clin. Nutr.*, 70, 405, 1999.

22. Heymsfield, S.B., Lichtman, S., Baumgartner, R.N., Wang, J., Kamen, Y., Aliprantis, A., and Pierson, Jr., R.N., Body composition of humans: comparison of two improved four-compartment models that differ in expense, technical complexity, and radiation exposure, *Am. J. Clin. Nutr.*, 52, 52, 1990.

23. Heymsfield, S.B. and Waki, M., Body composition in humans: advances in the development of multicompartment chemical models, *Nutr. Rev.*, 49, 97, 1991.

24. Lohman, T.G. and Going, S.B., Multicomponent Models in Body Composition Research: Opportunities and Pitfalls, in *Human Body Composition*, Ellis, K.J. and Eastman, J.D., Eds., Plenum Press, New York, 1993, p. 53.

25. Snead, D.B., Birge, S.J., and Kohrt, W.M., Age-related differences in body composition by hydrodensitometry and dual-energy X-ray absorptiometry, *J. Appl. Physiol.*, 74, 770, 1993.

26. Clasey, J.L., Kanaley, J.A., Wideman, L., Heymsfield, S.B., Teates, C.D., Gutgesell, M.E., Thorner, M.O., Hartman, M.L., and Weltman, A., Validity of methods of body composition assessment in young and older men and women, *J. Appl. Physiol.*, 86, 1728, 1999.

27. Salamone, L.M., Fuerst, T., Visser, M., Kern, M., Lang, T., Dockrell, M., Cauley, J.A., Nevitt, M., Tylavsky, F., and Lohman, T.G., Measurement of fat mass using DEXA: a validation study in elderly adults, *J. Appl. Physiol.*, 89, 345, 2000.

28. Ravaglia, G., Forti, P., Maioli, F., Boschi, F., Cicognani, A., and Gasbarrini, G., Measurement of body fat in healthy elderly men: a comparison of methods, *J. Gerontol. A Biol. Sci. Med. Sci.*, 54, M70, 1999.

29. Tataranni, P.A. and Ravussin, E., Use of dual-energy X-ray absorptiometry in obese individuals, *Am. J. Clin. Nutr.*, 62, 730, 1995.

30. Andreoli, A., Monteleone, M., Van Loan, M., Promenzio, L., Tarantino, U., and De Lorenzo, A., Effects of different sports on bone density and muscle mass in highly trained athletes, *Med. Sci. Sports Exerc.*, 33, 507, 2001.

31. Plowman, S.A., Drinkwater, B.L., and Horvath, S.M., Age and aerobic power in women: a longitudinal study, *J. Gerontol.*, 34, 512, 1979.

32. Hetland, M.L., Haarbo, J., and Christiansen, C., Regional body composition determined by dual-energy X-ray absorptiometry. Relation to training, sex hormones, and serum lipids in male long-distance runners, *Scand. J. Med. Sci. Sports*, 8, 102, 1998.

33. Ryan, A.S., Nicklas, B.J., and Elahi, D., A cross-sectional study on body composition and energy expenditure in women athletes during aging, *Am. J. Physiol.*, 271, E916, 1996.

34. Van Pelt, R.E., Davy, K.P., Stevenson, E.T., Wilson, T.M., Jones, P.P., Desouza, C.A., and Seals, D.R., Smaller differences in total and regional adiposity with age in women who regularly perform endurance exercise, *Am. J. Physiol.*, 275, E626, 1998.

35. Tanaka, H., Desouza, C.A., Jones, P.P., Stevenson, E.T., Davy, K.P., and Seals, D.R., Greater rate of decline in maximal aerobic capacity with age in physically active vs. sedentary healthy women, *J. Appl. Physiol.*, 83, 1947, 1997.

36. Madsen, K.L., Adams, W.C., and Van Loan, M.D., Effects of physical activity, body weight and composition, and muscular strength on bone density in young women, *Med. Sci. Sports Exerc.*, 30, 114, 1998.

37. Yataco, A.R., Busby-Whitehead, J., Drinkwater, D.T., and Katzel, L.I., Relationship of body composition and cardiovascular fitness to lipoprotein lipid profiles in master athletes and sedentary men, *Aging (Milano)*, 9, 88, 1997.

38. Seals, D.R., Allen, W.K., Hurley, B.F., Dalsky, G.P., Ehsani, A.A., and Hagberg, J.M., Elevated high-density lipoprotein cholesterol levels in older endurance athletes, *Am. J. Cardiol.*, 54, 390, 1984.

39. Northcote, R.J., Canning, G.C., Todd, I.C., and Ballantyne, D., Lipoprotein profiles of elite veteran endurance athletes, *Am. J. Cardiol.*, 61, 934, 1988.

40. Heath, G.W., Hagberg, J.M., Ehsani, A.A., and Holloszy, J.O., A physiological comparison of young and older endurance athletes, *J. Appl. Physiol.*, 51, 634, 1981.

41. McCole, S.D., Brown, M.D., Moore, G.E., Zmuda, J.M., Cwynar, J.D., and Hagberg, J.M., Enhanced cardiovascular hemodynamics in endurance-trained postmenopausal women athletes, *Med. Sci. Sports Exerc.*, 32, 1073, 2000.

42. Wells, C.L., Boorman, M.A., and Riggs, D.M., Effect of age and menopausal status on cardiorespiratory fitness in master women runners, *Med. Sci. Sports Exerc.*, 24, 1147, 1992.

43. Davy, K.P., Evans, S.L., Stevenson, E.T., and Seals, D.R., Adiposity and regional body fat distribution in physically active young and middle-aged women, *Int. J. Obesity Related Metab. Disorders*, 20, 777, 1996.

44. Wiswell, R.A., Jaque, S.V., Marcell, T.J., Hawkins, S.A., Tarpenning, K.M., Constantino, N., and Hyslop, D.M., Maximal aerobic power, lactate threshold, and running performance in master athletes, *Med. Sci. Sports Exerc.*, 32, 1165, 2000.

45. Kohrt, W.M., Malley, M.T., Dalsky, G.P., and Holloszy, J.O., Body composition of healthy sedentary and trained, young and older men and women, *Med. Sci. Sports Exerc.*, 24, 832, 1992.

46. Pollock, M.L., Gettman, L.R., Jackson, A., Ayres, J., Ward, A., and Linnerud, A.C., Body composition of elite class distance runners, *Ann. N.Y. Acad. Sci.*, 301, 361, 1977.

47. Pollock, M.L., Miller, H., Jr., S., and Wilmore, J., Physiological characteristics of champion American track athletes 40 to 75 years of age, *J. Gerontol.*, 29, 645, 1974.

48. Kavanagh, T. and Shephard, R.J., The effects of continued training on the aging process, *Ann. N.Y. Acad. Sci.*, 301, 656, 1977.

49. Proctor, D.N. and Joyner, M.J., Skeletal muscle mass and the reduction of VO$_2$max in trained older subjects, *J. Appl. Physiol.*, 82, 1411, 1977.

50. Reed, R.L., Yochum, K., Pearlmutter, L., Meredith, K.E., and Mooradian, A.D., The interrelationship between physical exercise, muscle strength and body adiposity in a healthy elderly population, *J. Am. Geriatr. Soc.*, 39, 1189, 1991.

51. Pollock, M.L., Foster, C., Knapp, D., Rod, J.L., and Schmidt, D.H., Effect of age and training on aerobic capacity and body composition of master athletes, *J. Appl. Physiol.*, 62, 725, 1987.

52. Trappe, S.W., Costill, D.L., Vukovich, M.D., Jones, J., and Melham, T., Aging among elite distance runners: a 22-yr longitudinal study, *J. Appl. Physiol.*, 80, 285, 1996.

53. Pollock, M.L., Mengelkoch, L.J., Graves, J.E., Lowenthal, D.T., Limacher, M.C., Foster, C., and Wilmore, J.H., Twenty-year follow-up of aerobic power and body composition of older track athletes, *J. Appl. Physiol.*, 82, 1508, 1997.

54. Marti, B., Knobloch, M., Riesen, W.F., and Howald, H., Fifteen-year changes in exercise, aerobic power, abdominal fat, and serum lipids in runners and controls, *Med. Sci. Sports Exerc.*, 23, 115, 1991.

55. Rogers, M.A., Hagberg, J.M., Martin, III, W.H., Ehsani, A.A., and Holloszy, J.O., Decline in VO$_2$max with aging in master athletes and sedentary men, *J. Appl. Physiol.*, 68, 2195, 1990.

56. Wilmore, J.H., Royce, J., Girandola, R.N., Katch, F.I., and Katch, V.L., Body composition changes with a 10-week program of jogging, *Med. Sci. Sports Exerc.*, 2, 113, 1970.

57. Hersey, W.C., III, Graves, J.E., Pollock, M.L., Gingerich, R., Shireman, R.B., Heath, G.W., Spierto, F., McCole, S.D., and Hagberg, J.M., Endurance exercise training improves body composition and plasma insulin responses in 70- to 79-year-old men and women, *Metabolism*, 43, 847, 1994.

58. Aldred, H.E., Hardman, A.E., and Taylor, S., Influence of 12 weeks of training by brisk walking on postprandial lipemia and insulinemia in sedentary middle-aged women, *Metabolism*, 44, 390, 1995.

59. Lehmann, R., Vokac, A., Niedermann, K., Agosti, K., and Spinas, G.A., Loss of abdominal fat and improvement of the cardiovascular risk profile by regular moderate exercise training in patients with NIDDM, *Diabetologia*, 38, 1313, 1995.

60. Despres, J.P., Bouchard, C., Tremblay, A., Savard, R., and Marcotte, M., Effects of aerobic training on fat distribution in male subjects, *Med. Sci. Sports Exerc.*, 17, 113, 1985.

61. Schwartz, R.S., Shuman, W.P., Larson, V., Cain, K.C., Fellingham, G.W., Beard, J.C., Kahn, S.E., Stratton, J.R., Cerqueira, M.D., and Abrass, I.B., The effect of intensive endurance exercise training on body fat distribution in young and older men, *Metabolism*, 40, 545, 1991.

62. Despres, J.P., Pouliot, M.C., Moorjani, S., Nadeau, A., Tremblay, A., Lupien, P.J., Theriault, G., and Bouchard, C., Loss of abdominal fat and metabolic response to exercise training in obese women, *Am. J. Physiol.*, 261, E159, 1991.

63. Kahn, S.E., Larson, V.G., Beard, J.C., Cain, K.C., Fellingham, G.W., Schwartz, R.S., Veith, R.C., Stratton, J.R., Cerqueira, M.D., and Abrass, I.B., Effect of exercise on insulin action, glucose tolerance, and insulin secretion in aging, *Am. J. Physiol.*, 258, E937, 1990.

64. Kirwan, J.P., Kohrt, W.M., Wojta, D.M., Bourey, R.E., and Holloszy, J.O., Endurance exercise training reduces glucose-stimulated insulin levels in 60- to 70-year-old men and women, *J. Gerontol.*, 48, M84, 1993.

65. Toth, M.J., Beckett, T., and Poehlman, E.T., Physical activity and the progressive change in body composition with aging: current evidence and research issues, *Med. Sci. Sports Exerc.*, 31, S590, 1999.

66. Glick, Z. and Kaufmann, N.A., Weight and skinfold thickness changes during a physical training course, *Med. Sci. Sports*, 8, 109, 1976.

67. Snyder, K.A., Donnelly, J.E., Jabosben, D.J., Hertner, G., and Jakicic, J.M., The effects of long-term, moderate intensity, intermittent exercise on aerobic capacity, body composition, blood lipids, insulin and glucose in overweight females, *Int. J. Obesity Related Metab. Disorders*, 21, 1180, 1997.

68. Laaksonen, D.E., Atalay, M., Niskanen, L.K., Mustonen, J., Sen, C.K., Lakka, T.A., and Uusitupa, M.I., Aerobic exercise and the lipid profile in type 1 diabetic men: a randomized controlled trial, *Med. Sci. Sports Exerc.*, 32, 1541, 2000.

69. Poirier, P., Catellier, C., Tremblay, A., and Nadeau, A., Role of body fat loss in the exercise-induced improvement of the plasma lipid profile in non-insulin-dependent diabetes mellitus, *Metabolism*, 45, 1383, 1996.

70. Schuit, A.J., Schouten, E.G., Miles, T.P., Evans, W.J., Saris, W.H., and Kok, F.J., The effect of six months training on weight, body fatness and serum lipids in apparently healthy elderly Dutch men and women, *Int. J. Obesity Related Metab. Disorders*, 22, 847, 1998.

71. Leon, A.S., Conrad, J., Hunninghake, D.B., and Serfass, R., Effects of a vigorous walking program on body composition, and carbohydrate and lipid metabolism of obese young men, *Am. J. Clin. Nutr.*, 32, 1776, 1979.

72. Lewis, S., Haskell, W.L., Wood, P.D., Manoogian, N., Bailey, J.E., and Pereira, M.B., Effects of physical activity on weight reduction in obese middle-aged women, *Am. J. Clin. Nutr.*, 29, 151, 1976.

73. Gwinup, G., Effect of exercise alone on the weight of obese women, *Arch. Intern. Med.*, 135, 676, 1975.

74. Kohrt, W.M., Obert, K.A., and Holloszy, J.O., Exercise training improves fat distribution patterns in 60- to 70-year-old men and women, *J. Gerontol.*, 47, M99, 1992.

75. Lee, L., Kumar, S., and Leong, L.C., The impact of five-month basic military training on the body weight and body fat of 197 moderately to severely obese Singaporean males aged 17 to 19 years, *Int. J. Obesity Related Metab. Disorders*, 18, 105, 1994.

76. Sopko, G., Leon, A.S., Jacobs, Jr., D.R., Foster, N., Moy, J., Kuba, K., Anderson, J.T., Casal, D., McNally, C., and Frantz, I., The effects of exercise and weight loss on plasma lipids in young obese men, *Metabolism*, 34, 227, 1985.

77. Ross, R., Dagnone, D., Jones, P.J., Smith, H., Paddags, A., Hudson, R., and Janssen, I., Reduction in obesity and related comorbid conditions after diet-induced weight loss or exercise-induced weight loss in men. A randomized, controlled trial, *Ann. Intern. Med.*, 133, 92, 2000.

78. Hadjiolova, I., Mintcheva, L., Dunev, S., Daleva, M., Handjiev, S., and Balabanski, L., Physical working capacity in obese women after an exercise programme for body weight reduction, *Int. J. Obesity*, 6, 405, 1982.

79. Miller, W.C., Koceja, D.M., and Hamilton, E.J., A meta-analysis of the past 25 years of weight loss research using diet, exercise or diet plus exercise intervention, *Int. J. Obesity Related Metab. Disorders*, 21, 941, 1997.

80. Westerterp, K.R., Obesity and physical activity, *Int. J. Obesity Related Metab. Disorders*, 23(suppl. 1), 59, 1999.

81. Walker, K.Z., Piers, L.S., Putt, R.S., Jones, J.A., and O'Dea, K., Effects of regular walking on cardiovascular risk factors and body composition in normoglycemic women and women with type 2 diabetes, *Diabetes Care*, 22, 555, 1999.

82. van Aggel-Leijssen, D.P., Saris, W.H., Wagenmakers, A.J., Hul, G.B., and van Baak, M.A., The effect of low-intensity exercise training on fat metabolism of obese women, *Obesity Res.*, 9, 86, 2001.

83. Ballor, D.L. and Keesey, R.E., A meta-analysis of the factors affecting exercise-induced changes in body mass, fat mass and fat-free mass in males and females, *Int. J. Obesity*, 15, 717, 1991.

84. Oscai, L.B., Mole, P.A., and Holloszy, J.O., Effects of exercise on cardiac weight and mitochondria in male and female rats, *Am. J. Physiol.*, 220, 1944, 1971.

85. Applegate, E.A., Upton, D.E., and Stern, J.S., Food intake, body composition and blood lipids following treadmill exercise in male and female rats, *Physiol. Behav.*, 28, 917, 1982.

86. Nance, D. et al., Sexually dimorphic effects of forced exercise on food intake and body weight in the rat, *Physiol. Behav.*, 19, 155, 1977.

87. Despres, J.P., Bouchard, C., Savard, R., Tremblay, A., Marcotte, M., and Theriault, G., The effect of a 20-week endurance training program on adipose-tissue morphology and lipolysis in men and women, *Metabolism*, 33, 235, 1984.

88. Depres, J.P. and Bouchard, C., Effects of aerobic training and heredity on body fatness and adipocyte lipolysis in humans, *J. Obesity Weight Regulation*, 3, 219, 1984.

89. Krotkiewski, M. and Bjorntorp, P., Muscle tissue in obesity with different distribution of adipose tissue. Effects of physical training, *Int. J. Obesity*, 10, 331, 1986.

90. Tremblay, A., Simoneau, J.A., and Bouchard, C., Impact of exercise intensity on body fatness and skeletal muscle metabolism, *Metabolism*, 43, 814, 1994.

91. Wilmore, J.H., Despres, J.P., Stanforth, P.R., Mandel, S., Rice, T., Gagnon, J., Leon, A.S., Rao, D., Skinner, J.S., and Bouchard, C., Alterations in body weight and composition consequent to 20 wk of endurance training: the HERITAGE family study, *Am. J. Clin. Nutr.*, 70, 346, 1999.

92. Westerterp, K.R., Alterations in energy balance with exercise, *Am. J. Clin. Nutr.*, 68, 970S, 1998.

93. Westerterp, K.R., Meijer, G.A., Janssen, E.M., Saris, W.H., and Ten Hoor, F., Long-term effect of physical activity on energy balance and body composition, *Br. J. Nutr.*, 68, 21, 1992.

94. Bouchard, C., Angelo, T., Jean-Pierre, D., Germain, T., Andre, N., Paul, L., Sital, M. Denia, P., and Guy, F., The response to exercise with constant energy intake in identical twins, *Obesity Res.*, 2, 400, 1994.

95. Perusse, L., Rice, T., Province, M.A., Gagnon, J., Leon, A.S., Skinner, J.S., Wilmore, J.H., Rao, D.C., and Bouchard, C., Familial aggregation of amount and distribution of subcutaneous fat and their responses to exercise training in the HERITAGE family study, *Obesity Res.*, 8, 140, 2000.

96.  Rice, T., Hong, Y., Perusse, L., Despres, J.P., Gagnon, J., Leon, A.S., Skinner, J.S., Wilmore, J.H., Bouchard, C., and Rao, D.C., Total body fat and abdominal visceral fat response to exercise training in the HERITAGE family study: evidence for major locus but no multifactorial effects, *Metabolism*, 48, 1278, 1999.

97.  Blumenthal, J.A., Sherwood, A., Gullette, E.C., Babyak, M., Waugh, R., Georgiades, A., Craighead, L.W., Tweedy, D., Feinglos, M., Appelbaum, M., Hayano, J., and Hinderliter, A., Exercise and weight loss reduce blood pressure in men and women with mild hypertension: effects on cardiovascular, metabolic, and hemodynamic functioning, *Arch. Intern. Med.*, 160, 1947, 2000.

98.  Weltman, A., Matter, S., and Stamford, B.A., Caloric restriction and/or mild exercise: effects on serum lipids and body composition, *Am. J Clin. Nutr.*, 33, 1002, 1980.

99.  Wood, P.D., Stefanick, M.L., Dreon, D.M., Frey-Hewitt, B., Garay, S.C., Williams, P.T., Superko, H.R., Fortmann, S.P., Albers, J.J., and Vranizan, K.M., Changes in plasma lipids and lipoproteins in overweight men during weight loss through dieting as compared with exercise, *N. Engl. J. Med.*, 319, 1173, 1988.

100.  Schwartz, R.S., The independent effects of dietary weight loss and aerobic training on high density lipoproteins and apolipoprotein A-I concentrations in obese men, *Metabolism*, 36, 165, 1987.

101.  Frey-Hewitt, B., Vranizan, K.M., Dreon, D.M., and Wood, P.D., The effect of weight loss by dieting or exercise on resting metabolic rate in overweight men, *Int. J. Obesity*, 14, 327, 1990.

102.  Abe, T., Kawakami, Y., Sugita, M., and Fukunaga, T., Relationship between training frequency and subcutaneous and visceral fat in women, *Med. Sci. Sports Exerc.*, 29, 1549, 1997.

103.  King, A.C., Haskell, W.L., Young, D.R., Oka, R.K., and Stefanick, M.L., Long-term effects of varying intensities and formats of physical activity on participation rates, fitness, and lipoproteins in men and women aged 50 to 65 years, *Circulation*, 91, 2596, 1995.

104.  Donnelly, J.E., Jacobsen, D.J., Heelan, K.S., Seip, R., and Smith, S., The effects of 18 months of intermittent vs. continuous exercise on aerobic capacity, body weight and composition, and metabolic fitness in previously sedentary, moderately obese females, *Int. J. Obesity Related Metab. Disorders*, 24, 566, 2000.

105.  Jakicic, J.M., Winters, C., Lang, W., and Wing, R.R., Effects of intermittent exercise and use of home exercise equipment on adherence, weight loss, and fitness in overweight women: a randomized trial, *JAMA*, 282, 1554, 1999.

106.  Dunn, A.L., Garcia, M.E., Marcus, B.H., Kampert, J.B., Kohl, H.W., and Blair, S.N., Six-month physical activity and fitness changes in Project Active, a randomized trial, *Med. Sci. Sports Exerc.*, 30, 1076, 1998.

107.  Dunn, A.L., Marcus, B.H., Kampert, J.B., Garcia, M.E., Kohl, III, H.W., and Blair, S.N., Comparison of lifestyle and structured interventions to increase physical activity and cardiorespiratory fitness: a randomized trial, *JAMA*, 281, 327, 1999.

108.  Pate, R.R., Pratt, M., Blair, S.N., Haskell, W.L., Macera, C.A., Bouchard, C., Buchner, D., Ettinger, W., Heath, G.W., and King, A.C., Physical activity and public health. A recommendation from the Centers for Disease Control and Prevention and the American College of Sports Medicine, *JAMA*, 273, 402, 1995.

# chapter seven

# Influence of endurance exercise on adipose tissue distribution

*Robert Ross, Ian Janssen, and Bente Stallknecht*

## Contents

0-8493-0460-1/02/$0.00+$1.50

## 7.1   Introduction

It is well known that adipose tissue is a heterogeneous organ characterized by marked differences in adipocyte metabolism, depending on anatomical location. Intra-abdominal or visceral adipocytes are more sensitive to adrenergic stimulation than abdominal subcutaneous adipocytes, which in turn are more sensitive than gluteal/femoral adipocytes. These differences are thought to be at least partially responsible for the gender differences in adipose tissue distribution and suggest that adipose tissue distribution may be influenced by various lifestyle and pharmacological interventions. Accordingly, as plasma catecholamine levels are elevated in response to exercise, it is not unreasonable to assume that regular exercise might alter adipose tissue distribution in a way that induces a preferential mobilization of abdominal adipose tissue. This would convey an important health benefit and reinforce the notion that exercise is a useful treatment strategy for obesity reduction.

The purpose of this chapter is twofold. The first is to review current knowledge with respect to variations in regional adipocyte metabolism in response to acute and chronic exercise. This will set the stage for the second objective, which is to review evidence that considers the effects of exercise training on adipose tissue distribution as measured by anthropometry and imaging modalities. In this way, we hope to bridge current knowledge with respect to the effects of exercise on adipocyte metabolism (*in vitro* and *in vivo* observations), with the known effects of exercise training on adipose tissue distribution. Finally, the issues and limitations upon which our summary observations were made are discussed, and recommendations for future research are provided.

## 7.2   Effects of exercise on adipose tissue metabolism

Over the last 10 years, the study of human adipose tissue metabolism has benefited from significant advances in research methodology. The microdialysis technique[1] and the combination of isotope methodology and catheterization[2,3] and fat biopsies[4,5] are among the technological advances that have helped characterize regional differences in adipose tissue metabolism *in vivo*. Indeed, these methodological advances together with conventional *in vitro* methodologies (fat biopsy) have firmly established the heterogeneity of human adipose tissue. Here, we provide a brief summary of the

metabolic differences that characterize adipose tissue. The intent is to provide a basis with which to consider the potential influence of exercise on the
metabolism of adipose tissue and thus its distribution.

## 7.2.1  Regional variation in adipose tissue metabolism at rest

In the basal state, lipolysis is higher or the same in femoral/gluteal compared
with subcutaneous abdominal adipose tissue in lean male and female subjects.[6-11] In obese subjects, lipolysis most often does not differ between subcutaneous abdominal and femoral adipose tissue.[9,12-14] Basal lipolysis is
higher in subcutaneous compared with intra-abdominal adipose tissue in
both lean and obese subjects.[15-18] Moreover, basal free fatty acid (FFA) release
from the upper body (including intra-abdominal adipose tissue) is higher
than from the lower body in both lean and obese subjects.[2,3,19,20] No gender
differences appear to be present with respect to regional variation in basal
lipolysis. However, black men and women have a higher basal lipolysis
compared with white men and women in both abdominal and femoral
adipose tissue.[10,14]

Lipolytic sensitivity toward catecholamines is higher in intra-abdominal
than in subcutaneous adipose tissue,[17,18,21] and generally higher in subcutaneous abdominal than in femoral/gluteal adipose tissue in both lean and
obese men and women.[6,22-24] Lipolytic sensitivity toward insulin (i.e., inhibition of lipolysis) is more pronounced in subcutaneous abdominal than in
femoral adipose tissue in lean and obese women,[25,26] and generally higher
in subcutaneous than in intra-abdominal adipose tissue in lean and obese
men and women.[16,19,21,27] Accordingly, it can be concluded that the "drive"
for lipolysis is higher in intra-abdominal compared with subcutaneous adipocytes during catecholamine/insulin stimulation. Also, during everyday
life (i.e., when the adipose tissue is influenced by varying concentrations of
catecholamines, insulin, and other hormones), lipid turnover is higher in
intra-abdominal than subcutaneous abdominal adipose tissue[28,29] and higher
in this tissue than in subcutaneous femoral adipose tissue.[4,5,30,31]

During acute exercise, adipose tissue lipolysis is stimulated by the
increase in sympathoadrenal activity and the decrease in insulin concentration.[32,33] From the previously mentioned studies, one would expect that
chronic exercise would induce a more pronounced stimulation of subcutaneous abdominal than femoral adipose tissue lipolysis. Intra-abdominal adipose tissue lipolysis would be expected to increase during acute exercise,
but the relative change in intra-abdominal compared with subcutaneous
adipose tissue is unclear.

## 7.2.2  Regional variation in adipose tissue metabolism
       during acute exercise

It is well established that *in vivo* adipose tissue lipolysis increases during
acute exercise;[34-37] however, few studies have examined the regional variation

in adipose tissue metabolism during exercise. For simplicity, the studies reviewed are considered according to the methodology employed to assess adipose tissue metabolism.

### 7.2.2.1   In vitro *studies*

The study of adipocyte metabolism *in vitro* relies on biopsy samples obtained from subcutaneous adipose tissue immediately post-exercise. Using this technique, it is observed that non-stimulated lipolysis is not changed by exercise in either subcutaneous abdominal or gluteal adipocytes in men or women (see Table 7.1).[38–41] In both men and women, the lipolytic responsiveness to β-agonist is increased in gluteal adipocytes post-exercise (Table 7.1).[39,40] The lipolytic responsiveness to norepinephrine,[40] epinephrine,[38] and post-adrenoceptor agents[40] was also increased in gluteal adipocytes from men after acute exercise. The lipolytic responsiveness to norepinephrine, however, was not changed by acute exercise in subcutaneous abdominal adipocytes from men or in abdominal or gluteal adipocytes from women (Table 7.1).[40] Also, acute exercise did not change the lipolytic responsiveness to β-agonist, norepinephrine, or epinephrine in subcutaneous abdominal adipocytes from women (Table 7.1).[41] Furthermore, acute exercise did not change lipolytic α-sensitivity or β- or α-receptor number in gluteal adipocytes in either men or women.[39,40] The implications of these observations are that gluteal adipocytes from men are more responsive to stimulation by all kinds of catecholamines after an acute bout of exercise; however, this is not the case for subcutaneous abdominal adipocytes from men or subcutaneous abdominal or gluteal adipocytes from women.

For obvious reasons, current knowledge regarding the effects of exercise on visceral adipocyte metabolism is based on animal studies. In female rats, basal and epinephrine-stimulated subcutaneous (inguinal) adipose tissue lipolysis, but not intra-abdominal (parametrial) adipose tissue lipolysis, is increased in response to 2 hours of continuous swimming.[42] Furthermore, adipose tissue lipoprotein lipase (LPL) activity is not influenced acutely by exercise, but 24 hours post-exercise, the intra-abdominal LPL activity was decreased.[42] In aggregate, these observations suggest that, in rats, intra-abdominal adipose tissue metabolism is unaltered by acute exercise. Whether these observations can be extrapolated to visceral adipocyte metabolism in humans is unclear.

### 7.2.2.2   *Catheterization studies*

In the 1970s, Ahlborg et al. published the first in a series of studies that employed the combination of isotope and catheterization techniques to characterize lipid turnover in different regions of the human body *in vivo*.[43] Specifically, the authors infused a radioactively labeled free fatty acid (FFA) intravenously and sampled blood from an artery, a femoral vein, and a hepatic vein.[43] Regional blood flow was measured by dye dilution technique. Lower-body (legs) and splanchnic FFA releases were calculated from measurements of arterial and venous FFA concentrations and specific activities of FFAs and regional blood flows.[43] Using this method, the authors report an increase in systemic, splanchnic, and lower-body rates of appearance of FFA in response to cycle exercise for 4 hr at 30% $VO_2$max in healthy, non-obese men.[43] The fractional contributions of FFA release from the lower body and the splanchnic area to systemic FFA turnover were approximately 20% and 7%, respectively, and did not change to any significant degree during the 4 hr of exercise.[43] In subsequent studies, Wahren et al.[44] observed an increase in systemic and splanchnic, but not in lower-body, rates of appearance of FFA in response to cycle exercise for 60 min at 45% $VO_2$max in healthy, non-obese men. However, in type I diabetic patients, they observed an increase in systemic and lower-body, but not in splanchnic, rates of appearance of FFA in response to the same exercise protocol.[44] Using a similar methodology, Burguera et al.[45] observed an increase in systemic and lower-body rates of appearance of FFA in response to cycle exercise performed for 90 min at 45% $VO_2$max with no difference between men and women. The fractional contribution of FFA release from the lower-body to systemic FFA turnover during the last 30 min of exercise was approximately 30% in men and 40% in women.[45]

Findings obtained by catheterization and *in vitro* studies are difficult to compare because catheterization studies examine changes in regional lipid metabolism during exercise and *in vitro* studies examine adipocytes after an acute bout of exercise. However, the catheterization studies reviewed indicate that acute exercise most often increases lipid turnover in all regions including the splanchnic region.

### 7.2.2.3 Microdialysis studies

First applied by Lönnroth et al.[1] in human adipose tissue and by Arner et al.[46] in rat adipose tissue, microdialysis is another method for studying adipose tissue metabolism *in vivo*. The microdialysis technique has been compared with *in vitro* measurements in isolated adipocytes in a group of obese subjects, and it was concluded that the two techniques provide similar and complementary information of adipose tissue metabolism.[47]

In 1990, Arner et al.[48] examined adrenergic regulation of lipolysis during cycle exercise for 30 min at 67% $VO_2$max in healthy, non-obese men and women (Table 7.1). Microdialysis probes were inserted into subcutaneous abdominal and gluteal adipose tissue, and changes in lipolysis were estimated from changes in dialysate glycerol concentration (i.e., with no calibration of microdialysis probes and not taking into account changes in adipose tissue blood flow and arterial glycerol concentrations).[48] The principal observation of this study was that lipolysis increased markedly more in subcutaneous abdominal than in gluteal adipose tissue during exercise, the difference between tissues being 50% in men and 300% in women.[48] The gender difference observed by Arner's group was confirmed by Hellström et al.,[49] who also observed a more pronounced exercise-induced increase in

Table 7.1  Influence of Acute and Chronic Exercise on Adipose Tissue Metabolism

| Ref. | Sex | BMI (kg/m²) [kg] | Exercise Stimulus | Basal Lipolysis | | Stimulated Lipolysis | |
|---|---|---|---|---|---|---|---|
| | | | | Abdominal Adipocytes | Femoral/ Gluteal Adipocytes | Abdominal Adipocytes | Femoral/ Gluteal Adipocytes |
| **Acute Exercise** | | | | | | | |
| *In vitro:* | | | | | | | |
| Savard et al.[38] | Young men | [66] | 88% heart rate max, 90 min | NR | — | NR | ↑ |
| Wahrenberg et al.[39] | Young men and women | 20.6 | 67% VO₂max, 30 min | NR | — | NR | ↑ |
| Wahrenberg et al.[40] | Young men | 22.8 | 67% VO₂max, 30 min | — | — | — | ↑ |
| | Young women | 22.7 | | — | — | — | ↑/— |
| Crampes et al.[41] | Young women | 21.3 | 60% heart rate reserve, 100 min | — | NR | — | NR |
| *Microdialysis:* | | | | | | | |
| Arner et al.[48] | Young men | 24.2 | 67% VO₂max, 30 min | ↑↑ | ↑ | NR | NR |
| | Young women | 21.5 | | ↑↑↑ | ↑ | NR | NR |
| Hellström et al.[49] | Young men | 23.5 | 67% VO₂max, 30 min | ↑↑↑ | NR | NR | NR |
| | Young women | 22.7 | | ↑↑↑ | NR | NR | NR |
| Horowitz et al.[11] | Young women | 21.2 | 50% VO₂max, 90 min | ↑↑↑ | — | NR | NR |
| Boschmann et al.[50] | Young men | 24.4 | 50% VO₂max, 60 min | ↑↑ | ↑↑↑ | NR | NR |
| | Young women | 22.2 | | ↑↑ | ↑↑↑ | NR | NR |
| **Chronic Training** | | | | | | | |
| *In vitro:* | | | | | | | |
| Mauriege et al.[7] | Young trained women | 21 | | Trained > sedentary | Trained ~ sedentary | Trained > sedentary | Trained ~ sedentary |
| | Young sedentary women | 22 | | | | | |

| Study | Subjects | | Protocol | | | | |
|---|---|---|---|---|---|---|---|
| Nicklas et al.[55] | Older women | [84] | 6-month diet | → | → | → | → |
| | | [81] | 6-month diet + aerobic exercise | — | — | — | — |
| *Microdialysis:* | | | | | | | |
| Horowitz et al.[24] | Young women | 21.2 | 12–14 weeks of aerobic exercise | — | — | — | — |
| Stallknecht et al.[59] | Young trained men | 22.5 | | Trained ~ sedentary | NR | Trained ~ sedentary | NR |
| | Young sedentary men | 22.8 | | | | | |
| Stich et al.[60] | Older men | 36.5 | 12 weeks of aerobic exercise | — | NR | ↑ | NR |
| Hickner et al.[26] | Lean trained women | [58] | | Sedentary obese > trained and sedentary lean | Sedentary obese > trained and sedentary lean | Trained and sedentary lean = sedentary obese (antilipolysis) | Trained and sedentary lean < sedentary obese (antilipolysis) |
| | Lean sedentary women | [61] | | | | | |
| | Obese sedentary women | [88] | | | | | |
| Stallknecht et al.[61] | Young trained men | 22.8 | | Trained ~ sedentary | NR | Trained < sedentary (antilipolysis) | NR |
| | Young sedentary men | 24.3 | | | | | |
| Hickner et al.[25] | Young women | [69] | 10 days of aerobic exercise | — | — | (antilipolysis) | (antilipolysis) |

*Note:* NR = not reported; — = no change; ↑ = increase; ↓ = decrease; ~ = equal to.

dialysate glycerol concentration in subcutaneous abdominal adipose tissue in women compared with men (Table 7.1).

Arner et al.[48] also examined the mechanisms that may account for the exercise-induced increase in adipose tissue lipolysis by adding sympathetic blockers to the ingoing microdialysis fluid.[48] In so doing, the authors determined that, whereas α-adrenergic mechanisms did not influence the exercise-induced increase in lipolysis in subcutaneous abdominal or gluteal adipose tissue, β-adrenergic mechanisms were important for the exercise-induced increase in lipolysis in subcutaneous abdominal adipose tissue (β-adrenergic mechanisms were not examined in gluteal adipose tissue).[48]

Horowitz et al.[11] examined lipolysis in subcutaneous abdominal and femoral adipose tissue in healthy, non-obese women during cycle exercise for 90 min at 50% $VO_2max$ (Table 7.1). Interstitial glycerol concentrations were measured by microdialysis and adipose tissue blood flow by $^{133}Xe$ washout technique; subsequently, adipose tissue lipolysis was calculated from these measurements and measurements of arterial glycerol concentrations.[11] The authors observed that subcutaneous abdominal adipose tissue lipolysis increased significantly during exercise, but that subcutaneous femoral adipose tissue lipolysis did not.[11] This study supports the study by Arner et al.[48] in that the exercise-induced increase in lipolysis is higher in subcutaneous abdominal than in lower-body subcutaneous adipose tissue in healthy, non-obese subjects.

Boschmann et al.[50] measured changes in dialysate glycerol concentration in subcutaneous abdominal and femoral adipose tissue during cycle exercise for 1 hr at 50% $VO_2max$ in healthy, non-obese men and women (Table 7.1). They found an exercise-induced increase in dialysate glycerol concentration of similar magnitude in both tissues and in both genders.[50] Furthermore, Boschmann et al.[50] estimated adipose tissue blood flow by microdialysis ethanol technique[51] and found a significant increase in blood flow in femoral and a nonsignificant increase in blood flow in subcutaneous abdominal adipose tissue during exercise in both sexes. The more pronounced exercise-induced increase in blood flow in femoral than in abdominal adipose tissue and similar exercise-induced increases in dialysate glycerol concentration indicated a higher exercise-induced lipolysis in femoral than in abdominal adipose tissue. This finding is in contrast to the finding by Arner et al.[48] A rationale that readily explains the discrepancy is unknown, but could be related to lower-body tissue examined (gluteal[48] and femoral,[50] respectively), time and intensity of the exercise protocol, or the position of the subject during the experiment because subjects sat upright on the cycle ergometer in the study by Arner et al.[48] and worked in a semisupine position in the study by Boschmann et al.[50] Subjects were of similar age and body mass index (BMI) in the two studies.[48,50]

### 7.2.2.4  *Adipose tissue blood flow*

Adipose tissue blood flow is an important parameter for the interpretation of studies examining adipose tissue metabolism *in vivo* because changes in venous or interstitial metabolite concentrations cannot be interpreted without knowledge of blood flow. Adipose tissue blood flow increases during acute exercise.[37,52] Regional variation in the exercise-induced increase in blood flow has been demonstrated because blood flow estimated by the [133]Xe washout technique increased 3 to 400% in subcutaneous lumbar adipose tissue and 700% in perirenal adipose tissue during cycle exercise of four 50-min sessions at 50% $VO_2$max separated by 10-min resting periods in young, healthy men.[53] As previously mentioned, blood flow estimated by microdialysis technique was found to increase significantly in femoral and nonsignificantly in subcutaneous abdominal adipose tissue during exercise.[50] In dogs, the regional variation in adipose tissue blood flow has been examined in greater detail by microsphere technique, and it was found that adipose tissue blood flow increased in all major adipose tissue depots during running exercise for 2 hr.[54] Exercise-induced increases were largest in perirenal, mesenteric, and pericardial depots (2.5- to 3-fold) and smallest in subcutaneous and parametrial depots.[54]

### 7.2.2.5 Conclusions

Few studies have examined regional variation in adipose tissue metabolism during acute exercise. An *in vitro* study found that basal lipolysis was not changed after acute exercise in either subcutaneous abdominal or gluteal adipocytes in either men or women. However, gluteal adipocytes, but not subcutaneous abdominal adipocytes, were more responsive to *in vitro* norepinephrine stimulation after exercise than before in men but not in women. Most microdialysis studies found that exercise stimulated *in vivo* lipolysis more in subcutaneous abdominal than in femoral/gluteal adipose tissue. Moreover, exercise of the same relative intensity increased subcutaneous abdominal adipose tissue lipolysis more in women than in men, as estimated by microdialysis. The apparent discrepancies between *in vitro* and microdialysis studies can probably be ascribed to the fact that the *in vivo* situation during exercise is more complex than the *in vitro* situation (i.e., changes in hormones, paracrine substances, and blood flow). Catheterization studies have shown that FFA release from the lower body contribute approximately 20% to systemic FFA turnover during low-intensity exercise and 30 to 40% during moderate-intensity exercise. The splanchnic area contributed approximately 7% to systemic FFA turnover during low-intensity exercise. Blood flow increased more in intra-abdominal than in subcutaneous adipose tissue during acute exercise.

## 7.2.3 Regional variation in adipose tissue metabolism in response to training

It is well known that training increases epinephrine-stimulated lipolysis and insulin-stimulated glucose uptake and their incorporation into triacylglycerol in adipocytes *in vitro*;[32,33] however, few studies have examined regional variation in adipose tissue metabolism in response to training.

### 7.2.3.1   In vitro *studies*

Mauriege et al.[7] studied adipocytes obtained using the biopsy technique from non-obese trained and sedentary premenopausal women and found that basal lipolysis expressed per cell as well as per cell surface area (i.e., corrected for variation in adipocyte size) was higher in trained than in sedentary women for both subcutaneous abdominal and femoral adipocytes (Table 7.1). Within each group, basal lipolysis expressed per cell was higher in femoral than in abdominal adipocytes, but when corrected for adipocyte size, differences disappeared.[7] Moreover, lipolytic responsiveness to β-agonist, epinephrine, and post-adrenoceptor agents and sensitivity to β-agonist were higher, and antilipolytic responsiveness to α-agonist and sensitivity to α-agonist were lower in subcutaneous abdominal adipocytes in endurance-trained women compared with sedentary women; however, training did not induce changes in femoral adipocytes.[7] In endurance-trained women, the lipolytic responsiveness to β-agonist and epinephrine was higher and the antilipolytic responsiveness to α-agonist was lower in subcutaneous abdominal than in femoral adipocytes, but no site differences were present in sedentary women.[7]

Nicklas et al.[55] studied the effects of diet alone vs. the combination of diet and training on subcutaneous abdominal and gluteal adipocytes in elderly, obese women (Table 7.1). In that study, 6 months of diet-induced weight loss decreased basal and epinephrine-stimulated lipolysis in subcutaneous abdominal and gluteal adipocytes.[55] However, the combination of diet and aerobic exercise performed 3 times per week at about 70% of $VO_2$max prevented the diet-induced decline in basal and epinephrine-stimulated lipolysis in both abdominal and gluteal adipocytes with no difference between tissues.[55]

Training decreased LPL-activity similarly in subcutaneous abdominal and femoral adipose tissue in both premenopausal, obese and non-obese women.[7,56] In non-obese women, LPL-activity expressed per cell as well as per cell surface area was higher in subcutaneous femoral than in abdominal adipose tissue,[7] whereas LPL-activity did not differ between tissues in obese women.[56]

The previously mentioned *in vitro* studies appear to suggest that training increases the lipolytic "drive" in subcutaneous abdominal adipocytes, whereas training decreases the uptake of lipid in both subcutaneous abdominal and femoral adipocytes. In other words, *in vitro* studies suggest that subcutaneous adipose tissue of trained subjects more easily lose lipid than gain it.

Swim training of rats for 4 weeks decreased LPL-activity per cell in intra-abdominal (parametrial and retroperitoneal), but not in subcutaneous (inguinal) adipose tissue; however, a further 2 weeks of training returned LPL-activities to pre-training levels.[57] Swim training of rats for 3 weeks abolished the pregnancy-induced increase in LPL-activity in intra-abdominal (parametrial and retroperitoneal), but not in subcutaneous (inguinal) adipose tissue.[58] Thus, although species differences may exist for the effect of training on LPL-activity in subcutaneous adipose tissue, rat studies suggest that training is also capable of decreasing LPL-activity in intra-abdominal adipose tissue.

### 7.2.3.2   Microdialysis studies

Horowitz et al.[11] studied lean, premenopausal women, who were endurance-trained for 12 to 14 weeks, and calculated subcutaneous abdominal and femoral adipose lipolysis from interstitial and arterial glycerol concentrations and adipose tissue blood flow (Table 7.1). Subjects were examined in the basal state and during 90 min of exercise performed at 50% of pretraining VO₂max; training did not change either basal or exercise-stimulated lipolysis at either site.[11] In lean men, Stallknecht et al.[59] found no effect of training on epinephrine-stimulated lipolysis in subcutaneous abdominal adipose tissue, whereas in obese men Stich et al.[60] observed an increased β-agonist-stimulated lipolysis in subcutaneous abdominal adipose tissue after training (Table 7.1).

Hickner et al.[26] estimated subcutaneous abdominal and femoral adipose tissue lipolysis from dialysate glycerol concentrations during a hyperinsulinemic, euglycemic clamp in non-obese endurance-trained, non-obese sedentary, and obese sedentary premenopausal women (Table 7.1). The percentage reduction in dialysate glycerol concentration during insulin infusion did not differ between groups in subcutaneous abdominal adipose tissue.[26] However, in femoral adipose tissue, dialysate glycerol concentration was reduced more in non-obese trained and sedentary women than in obese sedentary women during a low insulin concentration, indicating a higher insulin sensitivity in non-obese than in obese women.[26] Stallknecht et al.[61] compared endurance-trained and sedentary non-obese men during a hyperinsulinemic, euglycemic clamp and found an increased insulin-sensitivity in subcutaneous abdominal adipose tissue of trained subjects both with respect to inhibition of lipolysis and stimulation of glucose uptake (Table 7.1). The reason for the discrepancy is unknown but could be related to the gender of subjects or the degree of training.

Hickner et al.[25] also studied the effects of 10 days of endurance exercise on subcutaneous abdominal and femoral adipose tissue lipolysis from dialysate glycerol concentrations obtained during a hyperinsulinemic, euglycemic clamp in premenopausal women (Table 7.1). Exercise did not change basal or insulin-suppressed lipolysis in either subcutaneous abdominal or femoral adipose tissue. However, the whole-body rate of appearance of glycerol (estimated by isotopic technique) was suppressed more by insulin after instead of before training. The authors concluded that intra-abdominal adipose tissue or skeletal muscle may be the site of improved antilipolytic response to insulin after training.[25]

Swim training of rats increased basal and epinephrine-stimulated lipolysis per 100 g of tissue in both intra-abdominal (retroperitoneal, parametrial, and mesenteric) and subcutaneous adipose tissue.[62] Basal and epinephrine-stimulated interstitial glycerol concentrations were higher in intra-abdominal than in subcutaneous adipose tissue in both trained and sedentary rats, indicating a higher lipolysis in intra-abdominal than in subcutaneous adipose tissue.[62] Swim training of rats increased insulin-stimulated glucose uptake per 100 g of tissue similarly in intra-abdominal (retroperitoneal, parametrial, and mesenteric) and subcutaneous adipose tissue.[63] Swim training of rats increased basal,[62,63] epinephrine-stimulated,[62] and insulin-induced[63] blood flow per 100 g in both intra-abdominal and subcutaneous adipose tissue. Basal and insulin-induced blood flow was higher in mesenteric than in other adipose tissues.[63]

### 7.2.3.3  Conclusions

Few studies have examined regional variations in adipose tissue metabolism in response to training. In non-obese women, training increased *in vitro* lipolytic responsiveness and sensitivity to catecholamines and decreased *in vitro* antilipolytic responsiveness and sensitivity to α-agonist in subcutaneous abdominal adipocytes but not in femoral adipocytes. Training did not change exercise-stimulated lipolysis in either subcutaneous abdominal or femoral adipose tissue of non-obese women when evaluated by microdialysis. Insulin sensitivity with respect to inhibition of lipolysis was higher in non-obese, trained and non-obese, sedentary women than in obese, sedentary women in femoral adipose tissue, but not in subcutaneous abdominal adipose tissue when evaluated by microdialysis. These observations are restricted to white women. The influence of age, race, and gender is unclear.

## 7.3  Exercise training and adipose tissue distribution

From the previous discussion, it is apparent that human adipocytes are characterized by marked differences in metabolism, depending on anatomical location. Visceral adipocytes are more sensitive to adrenergic stimulation as compared to abdominal subcutaneous adipocytes, which in turn are more sensitive to adrenergic stimulation than gluteal/femoral adipocytes. Accordingly, because circulating catecholamine levels are elevated in response to exercise, it is reasonable to suggest that chronically performed exercise may induce a preferential reduction in abdominal obesity. Indeed, as reviewed here, Arner et al.[48] have shown that, during aerobic exercise in both sexes, a marked increase in the mobilization of lipids from abdominal subcutaneous adipose tissue occurs, whereas only a minor increase in lipolytic activity is observed in gluteal subcutaneous adipose tissue. Based on this premise, whether exercise training affects adipose tissue distribution is considered from two perspectives. First, does the addition of exercise to caloric restriction induce a greater reduction in abdominal and/or visceral adipose tissue by comparison to caloric restriction alone? Second, does exercise training with or without weight loss change adipose tissue distribution? In this section, the authors review the literature that considers these questions.

## 7.3.1 Diet alone vs. diet and exercise training

### 7.3.1.1 Observations using anthropometry

In weight-loss studies, abdominal obesity is commonly measured by either waist-to-hip circumference ratio (WHR) or waist circumference alone. Although waist circumference is a stronger correlate of changes in abdominal and visceral adipose tissue by comparison with WHR,[64,65] WHR is a useful method to determine the influence of a given perturbation on adipose tissue distribution. For example, reduction in WHR consequent to weight loss may indicate a greater reduction in abdominal adipose tissue compared with gluteal/femoral subcutaneous adipose tissue.

The influence of diet and exercise on adipose tissue distribution has received less attention compared with its effects on obesity per se. However, consistent with the observation that the addition of exercise training does not enhance diet-induced fat loss,[66,67] diet and exercise combined do not appear to enhance reductions in abdominal obesity (waist circumference) or adipose tissue distribution, or WHR, when compared with diet alone (see Table 7.2).[67-72] This might be expected given that, without exception, the addition of exercise training did not increase body weight loss or fat loss by comparison with diet alone. It is noted, however, that without exception the reduction in waist circumference is numerically greater in response to diet and exercise combined (Table 7.2). The relatively small cohort size in these studies suggests that they may be underpowered to determine true treatment differences. Finally, because these observations are based entirely on studies that employ white, overweight, and obese men and women, the potential influence of race is unknown.

### 7.3.1.2 Observations using imaging methods

The authors are aware of only three studies that consider whether diet and exercise training combined have effects on adipose tissue distribution that are different than diet alone (Table 7.2).[55,67,72] Consistent with the findings based on anthropometric variables, limited evidence suggests that the addition of moderate-intensity exercise training (50 to 75% of $VO_2max$) performed 3 to 5 times per week does not appear to augment the reduction in abdominal subcutaneous or visceral adipose tissue compared to diet alone in overweight and/or obese men[67] or women.[55,72] However, similar to diet-induced weight loss, a preferential reduction in visceral adipose tissue is observed in response to the combination of diet and exercise. For example, Ross et al.[67] and Janssen and Ross[72] observed that the relative reduction in visceral adipose tissue was ~11% greater than the corresponding reduction in abdominal subcutaneous adipose tissue in response to diet alone or the combination of diet and exercise in obese men and women.

As reviewed earlier, Nicklas et al.[55] considered the effects of exercise training on abdominal subcutaneous and gluteal adipocyte metabolism in addition to the measurement of abdominal subcutaneous adipose tissue. The authors observed that basal and epinephrine-stimulated lipolysis declined

Table 7.2 Influence of Diet Alone vs. Combination of Diet and Exercise Training on Adipose Tissue Distribution

| Ref. | Subjects Sex | BMI (kg/m²) [kg] | Treatment | Study Duration (months) | Weight Loss (kg) | VAT Loss [%] | ASAT Loss [%] | Reduction in WHR | Reduction in WC (cm) |
|---|---|---|---|---|---|---|---|---|---|
| **Anthropometry** | | | | | | | | | |
| Stefanick et al.[68] | Men | [84] | Control | 12 | +0.5 | NR | NR | 0.01 | NR |
| | | | Diet alone | | 2.8 | | | 0.02 | |
| | | | Diet + aerobic exercise | | 4.2 | | | 0.03 | |
| Stefanick et al.[68] | Older women | [70] | Control | 12 | +0.8 | NR | NR | 0.01 | NR |
| | | | Diet alone | | 2.7 | | | 0.01 | |
| | | | Diet + aerobic exercise | | 3.1 | | | 0.01 | |
| Dengel et al.[69] | Men | [84] | Control | 10 | +1.2 | NR | NR | No change | No change |
| | | [92] | Diet alone | | 7.6 | | | 0.00 | 8.0 |
| | | [94] | Diet + aerobic exercise | | 8.0 | | | 0.02 | 7.0 |
| Whatley et al.[70] | Women | 34 | Diet alone | 3 | 13.1 | NR | NR | 0.03 | NR |
| | | 36 | Diet + LV aerobic exercise | | 15.8 | | | 0.04 | |
| | | 35 | Diet + HV aerobic exercise | | 19.6 | | | 0.02 | |

| Study | Subjects | Reference | Group | N | | | | | |
|---|---|---|---|---|---|---|---|---|---|
| Wood et al.[71] | Men | [98] | Control | 12 | +1.7 | NR | NR | 0.00 | NR |
| | | | Diet alone | | 5.1 | | | 0.02 | |
| | | | Diet + aerobic exercise | | 8.7 | | | 0.04 | |
| Wood et al.[71] | Women | [75] | Control | 12 | +1.3 | NR | NR | 0.00 | NR |
| | | | Diet alone | | 4.1 | | | 0.01 | |
| | | | Diet + aerobic exercise | | 5.1 | | | 0.03 | |
| **Imaging** | | | | | | | | | |
| Janssen and Ross[72] | Women | 34 | Diet alone | 4 | 10.7 | 0.7 kg [31] | 1.4 kg [19] | 0.00 | 7.3 |
| | | 35 | Diet + aerobic exercise | | 11.5 | 0.7 kg [35] | 1.7 kg [24] | 0.02 | 9.0 |
| | | 33 | Diet + resistance exercise | | 10.9 | 0.4 kg [30] | 1.7 kg [28] | 0.03 | 10.6 |
| Nicklas et al.[55] | Older women | [74] | Diet alone | 6 | 9.8 | 21 cm² [14] | 77 cm² [17] | NR | NR |
| | | [74] | Diet + aerobic exercise | | 6.6 | 26 cm² [20] | 65 cm² [15] | | |
| Ross et al.[67] | Men | 32 | Diet alone | 4 | 11.4 | 1.5 L [32] | [21] | 0.03 | 8.5 |
| | | 33 | Diet + aerobic exercise | | 11.6 | 1.8 L [39] | [28] | 0.05 | 12.9 |
| | | 33 | Diet + resistance exercise | | 13.2 | 1.4 L [40] | [32] | 0.05 | 11.9 |

*Note:*  ASAT = abdominal subcutaneous adipose tissue; BMI = body mass index; HV = high-volume; LV = low-volume; NR = not reported; VAT = visceral adipose tissue; WC = waist circumference; WHR = waist-to-hip ratio.

in both abdominal and gluteal adipocytes within the diet-only group, but was unchanged in the diet-and-exercise group. The fact that exercise training prevented a decline in basal and epinephrine-stimulated lipolysis by a similar magnitude in both tissues reinforces the expectation that exercise training should be associated with a greater reduction in total adiposity and abdominal subcutaneous adipose tissue compared with diet alone. The basis for this argument is that acute exercise is associated with elevations in circulating levels of catecholamines. This was not observed by Nicklas et al.[55] and is not readily explained; however, it is noteworthy that body weight was reduced by an additional 30% in the diet-only group (Table 7.2), thus underscoring the challenge inherent to diet control in studies that employ free-living subjects.

Although the addition of exercise training to a program of energy restriction (diet) does not enhance the reduction in total abdominal adipose tissue, it is reported that the combination of diet and exercise results in a greater reduction in abdominal subcutaneous vs. peripheral (gluteal/femoral) subcutaneous adipose tissue (see Figure 7.1). Figure 7.1 illustrates that, in moderately obese men and women, the relative reduction in abdominal subcutaneous adipose tissue is greater than leg subcutaneous adipose tissue in response to diet and aerobic or resistance exercise, but not diet alone. This observation is consistent with the work of Arner et al., who reported that an acute bout of aerobic exercise is associated with a marked increase in the mobilization of lipids from abdominal subcutaneous adipose tissue, whereas only a minor increase in lipolytic activity is observed in gluteal subcutaneous adipose tissue.[48] Inasmuch as abdominal subcutaneous adipose tissue independently contributes to the increase in metabolic risk factors, particularly insulin resistance,[73,74] this observation suggests that the combination of diet and exercise may confer health benefits that are greater than diet alone. Clearly, these observations require confirmation in studies with larger cohorts of different ages and races.

## 7.3.2   Influence of exercise training with and without weight loss on adipose tissue distribution

### 7.3.2.1   Observations using anthropometry

Eleven controlled trials have considered whether exercise training with or without weight loss has an influence on abdominal obesity (waist circumference) or adipose tissue distribution (WHR) (see Table 7.3).[64,68,75–83] In general, training in the absence of weight loss is not associated with changes in either waist circumference or WHR. In contrast, for those studies that do observe an exercise-induced weight loss, abdominal obesity by waist circumference is significantly reduced by comparison with controls (Table 7.3).[64,79,81,82] A similar trend is observed for the noncontrolled studies (Table 7.3).[84–92] Whereas waist circumference is unchanged for those studies reporting no loss in weight or fat,[85–87] a modest reduction is observed in response to weight loss in the order of 2 kg.[88–91] In summary, observations based on

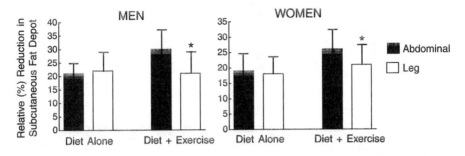

*Figure 7.1*    Relative reduction in abdominal (solid bars) and leg (open bars) subcutaneous adipose tissue in response to diet alone or the combination of diet plus
exercise in obese men (left) and premenopausal, obese women (right). Within both
genders, the relative reduction in abdominal and leg subcutaneous adipose tissue
was not different in response to diet alone. Within both genders, the relative reduction
in abdominal subcutaneous adipose tissue was greater than leg subcutaneous adipose tissue in response to diet plus exercise (*). Data are presented as group means
± SD. (Adapted from Ross, R. et al., *J. Appl. Physiol.*, 81, 2445, 1996, (men) and
Janssen, I. and Ross, R., *Int. J. Obesity*, 23, 1035, 1999, (women).)

anthropometry suggest that abdominal adipose tissue is reduced concurrent
with exercise-induced weight loss, but not in the absence of weight loss. The
same is not true for adipose tissue distribution measured by WHR. With a
single exception,[64] independent of gender, exercise-induced changes in WHR
with or without weight loss are not different from controls (Table 7.3). Thus,
it would appear that the mobilization of lipids as a consequence of aerobic-
type exercise training measured by anthropometry (WHR) is relatively uni-
form. Alternatively, it is possible that the WHR lacks the sensitivity to detect
subtle yet clinically significant changes in adipose tissue distribution. Again,
these observations are restricted to white men and women.

### 7.3.2.2    Observations using imaging methods

We are aware of four controlled[64,75,93,94] and six uncontrolled[84,85,95–98] trials that
report on the influence of exercise training on subcutaneous and visceral
adipose tissue distribution (see Table 7.4). For simplicity, we consider those
studies that report exercise with or without weight loss separately.

### 7.3.2.2.1    Exercise without weight loss.

Mourier et al.[75] observed large
reductions in both visceral (~48%) and abdominal subcutaneous adipose
tissue (~18%) in response to moderate exercise performed 3 times per week
for 8 weeks in men and women with type II diabetes. Although numerically
the reduction in visceral adipose tissue in this study was substantial in
comparison with subcutaneous adipose tissue, the authors did not report
whether the respective reductions were statistically different. Ross et al.[64]
observed a 16% reduction in visceral adipose tissue independent of any
change in abdominal subcutaneous or total adipose tissue in obese men who
performed daily (~60 min) aerobic exercise (brisk walking) for 3 months.

Table 7.3 Influence of Exercise Training on Fat Distribution Measured by Waist-to-Hip Ratio and Waist Circumference

| Ref. | Subjects | | Treatment | Study Duration (months) | Reduction in Weight (kg) | Reduction in WHR | Reduction in WC (cm) |
| | Sex | BMI (kg/m²) [kg] | | | | | |
| --- | --- | --- | --- | --- | --- | --- | --- |
| **Randomized, Controlled Trials** | | | | | | | |
| Ross et al.[64] | Men | 31 | Control group | 3 | 0.8 | 0.00 | 0.1 |
| | | 32 | Aerobic exercise | | 7.6[b] | 0.03[b] | 6.8[b] |
| Stefanick et al.[68] | Hyperlipidemic women | [~70] | Control group | 12 | +0.8 | 0.01 | NR |
| | | [~70] | Aerobic exercise | | 0.4 | 0.01 | |
| Stefanick et al.[68] | Hyperlipidemic men | [~84] | Control group | 12 | +0.5 | 0.01 | NR |
| | | [~84] | Aerobic exercise | | 0.6 | 0.01 | |
| Mourier et al.[75] | Diabetic men and women | 30 | Control group | 2 | 0.2 | 0.01 | 0.0 |
| | | 30 | Aerobic exercise | | 1.5 | 0.03 | 1.0 |
| Dengel et al.[76] | Older men | [90] | Control group | 10 | 0.2 | 0.00 | NR |
| | | [95] | Aerobic exercise | | 0.5 | 0.01 | |
| Binder et al.[77] | Older women | 25 | Control group | 12 | +0.6 | NR | +0.4 |
| | Older women | 25 | Aerobic exercise | | 1.2[a] | | 3.1[a] |
| Katzel et al.[78] | Older men | 30 | Control group | 9 | NS | NS | NS |
| | | 30 | Aerobic exercise | | NS | NS | NS |
| Lehmann et al.[79] | Diabetic men and women | 31 | Control group | 3 | 0.0 | 0.00 | 0.0 |
| | | 31 | Aerobic exercise | | 0.7 | 0.03[a] | 3.3[a] |
| Treuth et al.[80] | Older men | [75] | Control group | 4 | NS | NS | NS |
| | | [85] | Resistance exercise | | NS | 0.03 | +2.0 |
| Hellénius et al.[81] | Hyperlipidemic men | 25 | Control group | 6 | +0.3 (BMI) | 0.05 | 0.3 |
| | | 25 | Aerobic exercise | | 0.3 (BMI)[a] | 0.06 | 2.2[a] |

| Reference | Subgroup | n | Group | | | | |
|---|---|---|---|---|---|---|---|
| Kohrt et al.[82] | Older men | 25 | Control group | 10 | 0.2 | +0.02 | +0.4 |
| | Older men | 27 | Aerobic exercise | | 3.4[a] | 0.03 | 3.9[a] |
| | Older women | 24 | Control group | | +1.2 | 0.01 | 0.1 |
| | Older women | 25 | Aerobic exercise | | 1.8[a] | 0.00 | 2.6[a] |
| Ballor et al.[83] | Women | [73] | Control group | 2 | 0.4 | NR | +0.4 |
| | Women | [74] | Aerobic exercise | | 0.5 | | +0.6 |
| **Non-Randomized Trials** | | | | | | | |
| Wilmore et al.[84] | Men | 26 | Aerobic exercise | 5 | 0.4[a] | 0.01[a] | 1.0[a] |
| | Women | 25 | Aerobic exercise | | 0.1 | 0.01[a] | 0.9[a] |
| Thomas et al.[85] | Young women | 25 | Aerobic exercise | 6 | 0.6 | 0 | NS |
| Katzel et al.[86] | Men | 29 | Aerobic exercise | 9 | 0.1 | 0 | 0.5 |
| Fonong et al.[87] | Old men and women | ~25 | Aerobic exercise | 2 | 0.2 | NR | 2 |
| Gredigan et al.[88] | Women | 24 | High-intensity aerobic exercise | 3 | 0.7 | NR | ~1 |
| | Women | 26 | Low-intensity aerobic exercise | | 3.3 | | ~3[a] |
| Houmard et al.[89] | Men | 30 | Aerobic exercise | 3 | 2 | 0.02[a] | 4.3[a] |
| Schwartz et al.[90] | Young men | 26 | Aerobic exercise | 7 | 0.5 | 0.00 | 1.8[a] |
| | Older men | 26 | Aerobic exercise | | 2.5[a] | 0.02[a] | 3.2[a] |
| Andersson et al.[91] | Men | ~25 | Aerobic exercise | 3 | 2.0[a] | 0.01 | 2.9[a] |
| | Women | | Aerobic exercise | | 0.7 | 0.01 | 3.6[a] |
| Coon et al.[92] | Older men | 31 | Diet group | 9 | 11.0[a] | 0.02 | NR |
| | | 30 | Aerobic exercise (WWL) | | 0.2 | +0.02 | NR |

*Note:*   BMI = body mass index; NR = not reported; NS = nonsignificant change ($p > 0.05$); WC = waist circumference; WHR = waist-to-hip circumference ratio; WWL = without weight loss.

[a] Significant change within group ($p < 0.05$).

[b] Significantly different than change in control group ($p < 0.05$).

This is consistent with Thomas et al.,[85] who examined the effects of exercise training without weight loss in 17 non-obese, healthy women. In that study, the women performed supervised, aerobic-type exercise 3 days a week for 6 months. Despite no change in total and subcutaneous adipose tissue as measured by magnetic resonance imaging, the authors reported a 25% reduction in visceral adipose tissue. Taken together, these studies[64,75,84] suggest that aerobic exercise training without weight loss results in marked reductions in visceral adipose tissue, which are in general greater than the change in total or abdominal subcutaneous adipose tissue. In contrast to these observations, Poehlman et al.[93] reported that 6 months of either endurance or resistance exercise training does not reduce abdominal subcutaneous or visceral adipose tissue in young, premenopausal women. This finding was consistent with DiPietro et al.,[94] who, in older men and women, reported that 4 months of supervised aerobic exercise has no effect on abdominal subcutaneous or visceral adipose tissue. A rationale that readily explains the equivocal findings is unknown. However, in the Poehlman et al.[93] study the average pre-treatment visceral adipose tissue values for the exercise groups approximated 40 cm$^2$, a value that is about 200% below the values thought to be associated with metabolic risk.[99,100] Taken together, there is no consensus as to the effects of exercise training in the absence of weight loss on abdominal adipose tissue distribution.

Little is known regarding the effects of exercise training without weight loss on the distribution of abdominal subcutaneous vs. leg subcutaneous adipose tissue. The authors are aware of five studies that have reported data for abdominal subcutaneous and leg subcutaneous adipose tissue measured with imaging techniques (Table 7.4).[64,75,93,95,98] Table 7.4 reveals that thigh adipose tissue was reduced in three of the five studies, and abdominal subcutaneous adipose tissue was reduced in two of the five studies; however, few of these studies report whether the changes in leg and abdominal subcutaneous adipose tissue were different. Two studies of note are those of Mourier et al.[75] and Schwartz et al.[97] Despite no change in thigh subcutaneous adipose tissue, Mourier et al.[75] reported an 18% reduction in abdominal subcutaneous adipose tissue in response to 8 weeks of aerobic exercise training in diabetic men and women. In contrast, Schwartz et al.[97] reported that thigh subcutaneous adipose tissue was reduced to a greater extent than abdominal subcutaneous adipose tissue in response to 7 weeks of aerobic exercise training in young men. Taken together, there appears to be no consensus as to the effects of exercise training in the absence of weight loss on subcutaneous adipose tissue distribution.

*7.3.2.2.2 Exercise-induced weight loss.* In general, for the studies reported in Table 7.4, the subjects were asked to refrain from any change in dietary practice; thus, at least in theory, the observed weight loss was induced by the exercise regimen alone. It is apparent from Table 7.4 that few studies have examined the effects of exercise-induced weight loss on adipose tissue distribution. Schwartz et al.[97] reported marked reductions in both abdominal subcutaneous (~20%) and visceral (~25%) adipose tissue in response to aerobic-type exercise in older men despite very modest weight loss (2.5 kg).[97] Consistent with the findings of this study, Wilmore et al.[84] recently reported that 5 months of cycling exercise performed 3 times per week by 557 men and women varying widely in age, race, and adiposity resulted in significant but small reductions in visceral adipose tissue (~6%) in association with a minor change in body weight and total fat (<1 kg). Bouchard et al.[96] studied seven twin pairs who exercised on a stationary bicycle 6 days a week for 3 months such that 1000 kcal were expended each day. In that study, the authors prescribed an isocaloric diet to ensure that the negative energy balance was induced by exercise alone. The exercise program resulted in a 5-kg reduction in body weight that was associated with a 36% reduction in visceral and 27% reduction in abdominal subcutaneous adipose tissue. Unfortunately, very little is known regarding whether exercise-induced weight loss influences the ratio of visceral to abdominal subcutaneous adipose tissue. Put another way, whether exercise alters adipose tissue distribution by inducing a greater reduction in visceral vs. subcutaneous fat is unclear.[101]

Of the ten studies shown in Table 7.4, only one study considers whether exercise-induced weight loss is associated with a change in the ratio of visceral to abdominal subcutaneous adipose tissue.[64] In that study, Ross et al. compared the effects of equivalent diet- or exercise-induced weight loss on abdominal obesity.[64] The authors reported that a 7.5-kg reduction in body weight induced by diet or exercise was associated with substantial and similar reductions in abdominal subcutaneous (~17%) and visceral fat mass (~26%). Moreover, within both the diet and exercise groups, a significant reduction in the ratio of visceral to subcutaneous adipose tissue mass was observed, underscoring the notion that during periods of negative energy balance, a change in fat distribution favors a reduction in visceral adipose tissue independent of whether diet or exercise induces weight loss.[64,102,103] Furthermore, within that same study the authors reported that the relative reduction in abdominal subcutaneous adipose tissue was greater than leg subcutaneous adipose tissue in response to exercise-induced, but not diet-induced, weight loss (see Figure 7.2). A finding consistent with the previously noted observation that diet and exercise training combined induce a preferential reduction in abdominal subcutaneous compared with gluteal/femoral subcutaneous adipose tissue compared with diet alone. This latter observation is consistent with the findings of Schwartz et al.,[97] who report that exercise-induced weight loss in elderly men resulted in a reduction in abdominal subcutaneous adipose tissue that was greater than thigh adipose tissue (~20% vs. no change).[97] Together, these observations support the heterogeneity of adipocyte metabolism based on anatomical location discussed in the first section of this chapter.

Table 7.4  Influence of Exercise Training on Changes in Visceral, Abdominal and Thigh Subcutaneous Adipose Tissue

| Ref. | Subjects Sex | BMI (kg/m²) [kg] | Treatment | Study Duration (months) | Reduction in Weight (kg) | Reduction in Body Fat (kg) | Initial VAT (cm²) | Reduction in VAT (cm²) [%] | Reduction in ASAT (cm²) [%] | Reduction in TSAT (cm²) [%] |
|---|---|---|---|---|---|---|---|---|---|---|
| **Randomized, Controlled Trials** | | | | | | | | | | |
| Ross et al.[64] | Men | 31 | Control group | 3 | 0.8 | 0.6 | 198 | 0 [0] | [3] | [1] |
| | | 33 | Exercise (WL) | | 7.6[b] | 6.1[b] | 186 | 52 [28][b] | [18][b] | [14][b] |
| | | 32 | Exercise (WWL) | | 0.5 | 0.8 | 191 | 32 [16][b] | [6] | [4] |
| Poehlman et al.[93] | Young women | 22 | Control group | 6 | +1.0 | 0.0 | 36 | +4 [11] | NR | +3 [3] |
| | | 22 | Aerobic exercise | | +2.0 | +1.0 | 36 | 0 [0] | 0 | 8 [8] |
| | | 22 | Resistance exercise | | 0.0 | -1.0 | 40 | +1 [2] | 1 | 6 [6] |
| DiPietro et al.[94] | Older men and women | 27 | Control group | 4 | 0.0 | NR | 116 | 18 [13] | +20 [8] | NR |
| | | 27 | Aerobic exercise | | 1.0 | | 136 | 10 [9] | +11 [6] | |
| Mourier et al.[75] | Diabetic men and women | 30 | Control group | 2 | 0.2 | 0.8 | 139 | 5 [3] | 9 [3] | 2 [3] |

| Study | Group | N | Exercise | | | | | | |
|---|---|---|---|---|---|---|---|---|---|
| | | 30 | Aerobic exercise | 1.5 | 0.8 | 156 | 76 [48] | 41 [18]^b | 1 [2] |
| **Non-Randomized Trials** | | | | | | | | | |
| Thomas et al.[85] | Young women | 25 | Aerobic exercise | 0.6 | 1.9 L | NR | 0.4 L [25] | NR | NR |
| Wilmore et al.[84] | Men | 26 | Aerobic exercise | 0.4^a | 0.9^a | 91 | 6 [7]^a | 10 [5]^a | NR |
| | Women | 25 | Aerobic exercise | 0.1 | 0.5^a | 67 | 3 [5]^a | 8 [3]^a | |
| Treuth et al.[95] | Older women | 25 | Resistance exercise | 0.1 | 0.4 | 144 | 14 [10]^a | 17 [6] | 8 [6]^a |
| Bouchard et al.[96] | Young men | [82] | Aerobic exercise | 5.0^a | 5.0^a | 81 | 29 [36]^a | 67 [27]^a | NR |
| Schwartz et al.[97] | Young men | 26 | Aerobic exercise | 0.5 | 1.6 | 66 | 11 [17]^a | 21 [10]^a | 33 [21]^a |
| | Old men | 26 | Aerobic exercise | 2.5^a | 2.4^a | 144 | 35 [25]^a | 35 [20]^a | 0 [0] |
| Després et al.[98] | Young women | 34 | Aerobic exercise | 3.7^a | 4.6^a | 125 | 3 [3] | 60 [11]^a | 36 [8]^a |

*Note:* ASAT = abdominal subcutaneous adipose tissue; BMI = body mass index; L = liters; NR = not reported; TSAT = thigh subcutaneous adipose tissue; VAT = visceral adipose tissue; WL = weight loss; WWL = without weight loss.

^a Significant change within group ($p < 0.05$).

^b Significantly different than change in control group ($p < 0.05$).

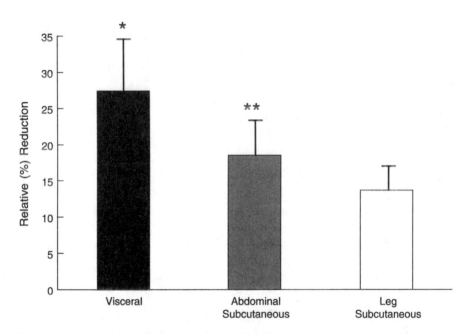

*Figure 7.2*    Relative reduction in visceral (solid bar), abdominal subcutaneous (gray bar), and leg subcutaneous (open bar) adipose tissue in response to exercise-induced weight loss in moderately obese men. The symbol * indicates that the relative reduction in visceral adipose tissue was greater than abdominal and leg subcutaneous adipose tissue; ** indicates that the relative reduction in abdominal subcutaneous adipose tissue was greater than leg subcutaneous adipose tissue. Data are presented as group means ± SD. (Adapted from Ross, R. et al., *Ann. Int. Med.*, 133, 92, 2000.)

## 7.4   Summary

The evidence reviewed supports the following summary observations:

1.   Acute exercise stimulates *in vivo* lipolysis, as estimated by microdialysis, more in subcutaneous abdominal adipose tissue than in femoral/gluteal adipose tissue. Moreover, exercise of the same relative intensity increases subcutaneous abdominal adipose tissue lipolysis more in women than in men. Catheterization studies show that FFA release from the lower body contributes approximately 20% to systemic FFA turnover during low-intensity exercise, whereas the splanchnic area contributes approximately 7%.

2.   On the basis of *in vitro* studies, exercise training increases the lipolytic "drive" in subcutaneous abdominal adipocytes, whereas training decreases the uptake of lipids in both subcutaneous abdominal and femoral adipocytes. This observation is restricted to white women because without exception, studies that have examined regional vari-

ation in adipose tissue metabolism in response to training have observed women.

3.  The combination of diet (caloric restriction) and exercise training does not influence abdominal obesity (waist circumference) or adipose tissue distribution (WHR) compared with diet alone. This observation remains true for abdominal subcutaneous and visceral adipose tissue. However, in comparison with diet alone, the combination of diet and exercise training is associated with a preferential reduction in abdominal subcutaneous vs. leg subcutaneous adipose tissue.

4.  Aerobic exercise training in the absence of weight loss is not associated with a reduction in abdominal obesity measured by waist circumference or adipose tissue distribution measured by WHR. Whether or not exercise training without weight loss is associated with significant reductions in adipose tissue distribution measured using imaging modalities is unclear.

5.  Exercise-induced weight loss is associated with reductions in abdominal obesity (waist circumference) but not adipose tissue distribution (WHR), as measured by anthropometry. Exercise-induced weight loss is associated with marked reductions in abdominal subcutaneous and visceral adipose tissue. Moreover, exercise-induced weight loss is also associated with a preferential reduction in abdominal subcutaneous vs. leg subcutaneous adipose tissue.

## 7.5   Issues and limitations

Absent from the literature are studies that consider simultaneously the effects of exercise training on adipose tissue metabolism and distribution. Moreover, given the acknowledged importance of abdominal obesity as an independent predictor of morbidity and mortality,[104–106] it is striking how few studies consider whether exercise training alone is an effective strategy for altering adipose tissue distribution. Nevertheless, available evidence suggests that exercise-induced weight loss is associated with a concomitant reduction in abdominal subcutaneous and visceral obesity. Limited evidence also supports the notion that the relative reduction in abdominal subcutaneous adipose tissue is greater than leg adipose tissue, and that adipose tissue distribution is altered in response to exercise training. Although the independent contribution of abdominal subcutaneous and visceral adipose tissue toward metabolic risk remains to be determined,[107] the fact that both depots are preferentially reduced in response to exercise training underscores the notion that exercise is a useful treatment strategy for obesity reduction. Indeed, at least three reports[64,75,85] suggest that exercise-induced reductions in visceral adipose tissue are related to concurrent reductions in insulin resistance independent of a change in abdominal subcutaneous or total adiposity.

The conclusions of this chapter are based in large measure on studies that employ middle-aged white men and women; thus, the influence of race is unknown. This is surprising given that, for example, for a given level of adiposity, blacks have less visceral adipose tissue than their white counterparts.[108,109] It is clear that additional studies are warranted that would consider potential differences in adipocyte metabolism and whether or not exercise-induced weight loss is influenced by race.

Determination of whether adipose tissue distribution is altered in response to exercise training requires obtaining both whole-body and regional measurements of adipose tissue distribution. Although not generally feasible, these measurements would ideally be obtained using either imaging or dual energy X-ray absorptiometry techniques. Acquisition of whole-body and regional measurements of adipose tissue distribution would permit the researcher to identify the separate contributions of, for example, abdominal vs. lower-body adipose tissue. Traditionally, determination of differences in regional obesity entailed comparisons of abdominal vs. whole-body adiposity. This analysis is confounded by the inclusion of abdominal adipose tissue in the whole-body measurement.

## 7.6   Conclusion

The purpose of this chapter was to bridge current knowledge with respect to the effects of exercise on adipocyte metabolism and adipose tissue distribution. Available evidence supports the view that in white men and women, exercise stimulates *in vivo* lipolysis more in subcutaneous abdominal adipose tissue than in femoral/gluteal adipose tissue. This is consistent with limited evidence suggesting that exercise-induced weight loss alters adipose tissue distribution in a way that induces a preferential mobilization of abdominal adipose tissue. Although the need for rigorously controlled trials that consider the effects of exercise training on adipose tissue distribution is apparent, current knowledge supports the view that exercise conveys an important health benefit and is a useful treatment strategy for obesity reduction.

## References

1. Lönnroth, P., Jansson, P.A., and Smith, U., A microdialysis method allowing characterization of intercellular water space in humans, *Am. J. Physiol.*, 253, E228, 1987.
2. Martin, M.L. and Jensen, M.D., Effects of body fat distribution on regional lipolysis in obesity, *J. Clin. Invest.*, 88, 609, 1991.
3. Jensen, M.D. et al., Effects of epinephrine on regional free fatty acid and energy metabolism in men and women, *Am. J. Physiol.*, 270, E259, 1996.
4. Mårin, P. et al., Glucose uptake in human adipose tissue, *Metabolism*, 36, 1154, 1987.

5. Mårin, P., Oden, B., and Björntorp, P., Assimilation and mobilization of trig-lycerides in subcutaneous abdominal and femoral adipose tissue in vivo in men: effects of androgens, *J. Clin. Endocrinol. Metab.*, 80, 239, 1995.
6. Wahrenberg, H., Lönnqvist, F., and Arner, P., Mechanisms underlying regional differences in lipolysis in human adipose tissue, *J. Clin. Invest.*, 84, 458, 1989.
7. Mauriege, P. et al., Regional differences in adipose tissue metabolism between sedentary and endurance-trained women, *Am. J. Physiol. Endocrinol. Metab.*, 273, E497, 1997.
8. Rebuffe-Scrive, M. et al., Fat cell metabolism in different regions in women. Effect of menstrual cycle, pregnancy, and lactation, *J. Clin. Invest.*, 75, 1973, 1985.
9. Jansson, P.A. et al., Glycerol production in subcutaneous adipose tissue in lean and obese humans, *J. Clin. Invest.*, 89, 1610, 1992.
10. Van der Merwe, M.T. et al., Lactate and glycerol release from subcutaneous adipose tissue in black and white lean men, *J. Clin. Endocrinol. Metab.*, 84, 2888, 1999.
11. Horowitz, J.F. et al., Effect of endurance training on lipid metabolism in women: a potential role for PPARα in the metabolic response to training, *Am. J. Physiol. Endocrinol. Metab.*, 279, E348, 2000.
12. Bolinder, J. et al., Site differences in insulin receptor binding and insulin action in subcutaneous fat of obese females, *J. Clin. Endocrinol. Metab.*, 57, 455, 1983.
13. Leibel, R.L. and Hirsch, J., Site- and sex-related differences in adrenoreceptor status of human adipose tissue, *J. Clin. Endocrinol. Metab.*, 64, 1205, 1987.
14. Van der Merwe, M.T. et al., Lactate and glycerol release from the subcutaneous adipose tissue of obese urban women from South Africa: important metabolic implications, *J. Clin. Endocrinol. Metab.*, 83, 4084, 1998.
15. Östman, J. et al., Regional differences in the control of lipolysis in human adipose tissue, *Metabolism*, 28, 1198, 1979.
16. Bolinder, J. et al., Differences at the receptor and postreceptor levels between human omental and subcutaneous adipose tissue in the action of insulin on lipolysis, *Diabetes*, 32, 117, 1983.
17. Hellmér, J. et al., Mechanisms for differences in lipolysis between human subcutaneous and omental fat cells, *J. Clin. Endocrinol. Metab.*, 75, 15, 1992.
18. Hoffstedt, J. et al., Variation in adrenergic regulation of lipolysis between omental and subcutaneous adipocytes from obese and non-obese men, *J. Lipid Res.*, 38, 795, 1997.
19. Meek, S.E., Nair, K.S., and Jensen, M.D., Insulin regulation of regional free fatty acid metabolism, *Diabetes*, 48, 10, 1999.
20. Jensen, M.D. and Johnson, C.M., Contribution of leg and splanchnic free fatty acid (FFA) kinetics to postabsorptive FFA flux in men and women, *Metabolism*, 45, 662, 1996.
21. Richelsen, B. et al., Regional differences in triglyceride breakdown in human adipose tissue: effects of catecholamines, insulin, and prostaglandin E2, *Metabolism*, 40, 990, 1991.
22. Mauriege, P. et al., Regional variation in adipose tissue lipolysis in lean and obese men, *J. Lipid Res.*, 32, 1625, 1991.
23. Mauriege, P. et al., Regional and gender variations in adipose tissue lipolysis in response to weight loss, *J. Lipid Res.*, 40, 1559, 1999.

24. Horowitz, J.F. and Klein, S., Whole-body and abdominal lipolytic sensitivity to epinephrine is suppressed in upper-body obese women, *Am. J. Physiol. Endocrinol. Metab.*, 278, E1144, 2000.
25. Hickner, R.C. et al., Effects of 10 days of endurance exercise training on the suppression of whole body and regional lipolysis by insulin, *J. Clin. Endocrinol. Metab.*, 85, 1498, 2000.
26. Hickner, R.C. et al., Suppression of whole-body and regional lipolysis by insulin: effects of obesity and exercise, *J. Clin. Endocrinol. Metab.*, 84, 3886, 1999.
27. Zierath, J.R. et al., Regional difference in insulin inhibition of non-esterified fatty acid release from human adipocytes: relation to insulin receptor phosphorylation and intracellular signalling through the insulin receptor substrate-1 pathway, *Diabetologia*, 41, 1343, 1998.
28. Mårin, P. et al., The morphology and metabolism of intra-abdominal adipose tissue in men, *Metabolism*, 41, 1242, 1992.
29. Mårin, P. et al., Assimilation of triglycerides in subcutaneous and intra-abdominal adipose tissues in vivo in men: effects of testosterone, *J. Clin. Endocrinol. Metab.*, 81, 1018, 1996.
30. Mårin, P., Rebuffe-Scrive, M., and Björntorp, P., Uptake of triglyceride fatty acids in adipose tissue in vivo in man, *Eur. J. Clin. Invest.*, 20, 158, 1990.
31. Mårin, P. et al., Uptake of glucose carbon in muscle glycogen and adipose tissue triglycerides in vivo in humans, *Am. J. Physiol.*, 263, E473, 1992.
32. Nicklas, B.J., Effects of endurance exercise on adipose tissue metabolism, *Exerc. Sport Sci. Rev.*, 25, 77, 1997.
33. Martin, W.H., Effects of acute and chronic exercise on fat metabolism, *Exerc. Sport Sci. Rev.*, 24, 203, 1996.
34. Bülow, J., Simonsen, L., and Madsen, J., Effects of exercise and glucose ingestion on adipose tissue metabolism, in *Integration of Medical and Sports Sciences*, Y. Sato, J. Poortmans, I. Hashimoto, and Y. Oshida, Eds., Karger, Basel, 1992, pp. 329–335.
35. Ranneries, C. et al., Fat metabolism in formerly obese women, *Am. J. Physiol.*, 274, E155, 1998.
36. Hodgetts, V. et al., Factors controlling fat mobilization from human subcutaneous adipose tissue during exercise, *J. Appl. Physiol.*, 71, 445, 1991.
37. Mulla, N.A., Simonsen, L., and Bülow, J., Post-exercise adipose tissue and skeletal muscle lipid metabolism in humans: the effects of exercise intensity, *J. Physiol. Lond.*, 524(part 3), 919, 2000.
38. Savard, R. et al., Acute effects of endurance exercise on human adipose tissue metabolism, *Metabolism*, 36, 480, 1987.
39. Wahrenberg, H. et al., Acute adaptation in adrenergic control of lipolysis during physical exercise in humans, *Am. J. Physiol.*, 253, E383, 1987.
40. Wahrenberg, H., Bolinder, J., and Arner, P., Adrenergic regulation of lipolysis in human fat cells during exercise, *Eur. J. Clin. Invest.*, 21, 534, 1991.
41. Crampes, F. et al., Lack of desensitization of catecholamine-induced lipolysis in fat cells from trained and sedentary women after physical exercise, *J. Clin. Endocrinol. Metab.*, 67, 1011, 1988.
42. Savard, R. et al., Site-specific effects of acute exercise on muscle and adipose tissue metabolism in sedentary female rats, *Physiol. Behav.*, 43, 65, 1988.
43. Ahlborg, G. et al., Substrate turnover during prolonged exercise in man. Splanchnic and leg metabolism of glucose, free fatty acids, and amino acids, *J. Clin. Invest.*, 53, 1080, 1974.

44. Wahren, J. et al., Turnover and splanchnic metabolism of free fatty acids and ketones in insulin-dependent diabetics at rest and in response to exercise, *J. Clin. Invest.*, 73, 1367, 1984.
45. Burguera, B. et al., Leg free fatty acid kinetics during exercise in men and women, *Am. J. Physiol. Endocrinol. Metab.*, 278, E113, 2000.
46. Arner, P. et al., Microdialysis of adipose tissue and blood for in vivo lipolysis studies, *Am. J. Physiol.*, 255, E737, 1988.
47. Kolehmainen, M. et al., Concordance of in vivo microdialysis and in vitro techniques in the studies of adipose tissue metabolism, *Int. J. Obesity*, 24, 1426, 2000.
48. Arner, P. et al., Adrenergic regulation of lipolysis in situ at rest and during exercise, *J. Clin. Invest.*, 85, 893, 1990.
49. Hellström, L., Blaak, E., and Hagström-Toft, E., Gender differences in adrenergic regulation of lipid mobilization during exercise, *Int. J. Sports Med.*, 17, 439, 1996.
50. Boschmann, M. et al., Physical activity shows differences in the effect of fat metabolism on men and women: results of a microdialysis study, *Forschende Komplementarmedizin*, 6, 52, 1999.
51. Hickner, R.C., Microdialysis in skeletal muscle, in *Development and Application of the Microdialysis Ethanol Technique*, Department of Physiology and Pharmacology, Division of Physiology, The Karolinska Institute, Stockholm, Sweden, 1995, pp. 1–67.
52. Bülow, J. and Madsen, J., Adipose tissue blood flow during prolonged, heavy exercise, *Pflüg. Arch.*, 363, 231, 1976.
53. Bülow, J. and Madsen, J., Human adipose tissue blood flow during prolonged exercise II, *Pflüg. Arch.*, 376, 41, 1978.
54. Bülow, J. and Tøndevold, E., Blood flow in different adipose tissue depots during prolonged exercise in dogs, *Pflüg. Arch.*, 392, 235, 1982.
55. Nicklas, B.J., Rogus, E.M., and Goldberg, A.P., Exercise blunts declines in lipolysis and fat oxidation after dietary-induced weight loss in obese older women, *Am. J. Physiol. Endocrinol. Metab.*, 273, E149, 1997.
56. Lamarche, B. et al., Evidence for a role of insulin in the regulation of abdominal adipose tissue lipoprotein lipase response to exercise training in obese women, *Int. J. Obesity*, 17, 255, 1993.
57. Savard, R. and Greenwood, M.R., Site-specific adipose tissue LPL responses to endurance training in female lean Zucker rats, *J. Appl. Physiol.*, 65, 693, 1988.
58. Savard, R., Palmer, J.E., and Greenwood, M.R., Effects of exercise training on regional adipose tissue metabolism in pregnant rats, *Am. J. Physiol.*, 250, R837, 1986.
59. Stallknecht, B. et al., Effect of training on epinephrine-stimulated lipolysis determined by microdialysis in human adipose tissue, *Am. J. Physiol.*, 269, E1059, 1995.
60. Stich, V. et al., Endurance training increases the beta-adrenergic lipolytic response in subcutaneous adipose tissue in obese subjects, *Int. J. Obesity*, 23, 374, 1999.
61. Stallknecht, B. et al., Effect of training on insulin sensitivity of glucose uptake and lipolysis in human adipose tissue, *Am. J. Physiol. Endocrinol. Metab.*, 279, E376, 2000.
62. Enevoldsen, L.H. et al., Effect of exercise training on in vivo lipolysis in intra-abdominal adipose tissue in rats, *Am. J. Physiol. Endocrinol. Metab.*, 279, E585, 2000.

63. Enevoldsen, L.H. et al., Effect of exercise training on in vivo insulin-stimulated glucose uptake in intra-abdominal adipose tissue in rats, *Am. J. Physiol. Endocrinol. Metab.*, 278, E25, 2000.

64. Ross, R. et al., Reduction in obesity and related comorbid conditions after diet-induced weight loss or exercise-induced weight loss in men: a randomized controlled trail, *Ann. Int. Med.*, 133, 92, 2000.

65. Kamel, E.G., McNeill, G., and Van Wijk, M.C.W., Change in intra-abdominal adipose tissue volume during weight loss in obese men and women: correlation between magnetic resonance imaging and anthropometric measurements, *Int. J. Obesity*, 24, 607, 2000.

66. Miller, W.C., Koceja, D.M., and Hamilton, E.J., A meta-analysis of the past 25 years of weight loss research using diet, exercise or diet plus exercise intervention, *Int. J. Obesity*, 21, 941, 1997.

67. Ross, R. et al., Influence of diet and exercise on skeletal muscle and visceral adipose tissue in men, *J. Appl. Physiol.*, 81, 2445, 1996.

68. Stefanick, M.L. et al., Effects of diet and exercise in men and postmenopausal women with low levels of HDL cholesterol and high levels of LDL cholesterol, *N. Engl. J. Med.*, 339, 12, 1998.

69. Dengel, D.R. et al., Distinct effects of aerobic exercise training and weight loss on glucose homeostasis in obese sedentary men, *J. Appl. Physiol.*, 81, 318, 1996.

70. Whatley, J.E. et al., Does the amount of endurance exercise in combination with weight training and a very-low-energy diet affect resting metabolic rate and body composition? *Am. J. Clin. Nutr.*, 59, 1088, 1994.

71. Wood, P.D. et al., The effects on plasma lipoproteins of a prudent weight-reducing diet, with or without exercise, in overweight men and women, *N. Engl. J. Med.*, 325, 461, 1991.

72. Janssen, I. and Ross, R., Effects of sex on the change in visceral, subcutaneous adipose tissue and skeletal muscle in response to weight loss, *Int. J. Obesity*, 23, 1035, 1999.

73. Goodpaster, B.H. et al., Subcutaneous abdominal fat and thigh muscle composition predict insulin sensitivity independently of visceral fat, *Diabetes*, 46, 1579, 1997.

74. Abate, N. et al., Relationship of generalized and regional adiposity to insulin sensitivity in men, *J. Clin. Invest.*, 96, 88, 1995.

75. Mourier, A. et al., Mobilization of visceral adipose tissue related to the improvement in insulin sensitivity in response to physical training in NIDDM, *Diabetes Care*, 20, 385, 1997.

76. Dengel, D.R. et al., Comparable effects of diet and exercise on body composition and lipoproteins in older men, *Med. Sci. Sports Exerc.*, 26, 1307, 1994.

77. Binder, E.F., Birge, S.J., and Kohrt, W.M., Effects of endurance exercise and hormone replacement therapy on serum lipids in older women, *J. Am. Geriatr. Soc.*, 44, 231, 1996.

78. Katzel, L.I. et al., Effects of weight loss vs. aerobic exercise training on risk factors for coronary disease in healthy, obese, middle-aged and older men, *JAMA*, 274, 1915, 1995.

79. Lehmann, R. et al., Loss of abdominal fat and improvement in the cardiovascular risk profile by regular moderate exercise training in patients with NID-DM, *Diabetologia*, 38, 1313, 1995.

80. Treuth, M.S. et al., Effects of strength training on total and regional body composition in older men, *J. Appl. Physiol.*, 77, 614, 1994.

81. Hellénius, M.L. et al., Diet and exercise are equally effective in reducing risk for cardiovascular disease. Results of a randomized controlled study in men with slightly to moderately elevated cardiovascular risk factors, *Atherosclerosis*, 103, 81, 1993.

82. Kohrt, W.M., Obert, K.A., and Holloszy, J.O., Exercise training improves fat distribution patterns in 60- to 70-year-old men and women, *J. Gerontol.*, 47, M99, 1992.

83. Ballor, D.L. et al., Resistance weight training during caloric restriction enhances lean body weight maintenance, *Am. J. Clin. Nutr.*, 47, 19, 1988.

84. Wilmore, J.H. et al., Alterations in body weight and composition consequent to 20 wk of endurance training: the HERITAGE Family Study, *Am. J. Clin. Nutr.*, 70, 346, 1999.

85. Thomas, E.L. et al., Preferential loss of visceral fat following aerobic exercise, measured by magnetic resonance imaging, *Lipids*, 35, 769, 2000.

86. Katzel, L.I. et al., Sequential effects of aerobic exercise training and weight loss on risk factors for coronary heart disease in healthy, obese middle-aged older men, *Metabolism*, 46, 1441, 1997.

87. Fonong, T. et al., Relationship between physical activity and HDL-cholesterol in healthy older men and women: a cross-sectional and exercise intervention study, *Atherosclerosis*, 127, 177, 1996.

88. Gredigan, M.A. et al., Exercise intensity does not effect body composition change in untrained, moderately overfat women, *J. Am. Diet. Assoc.*, 95, 661, 1995.

89. Houmard, J.A. et al., Effects of exercise training on absolute and relative measurements of regional adiposity, *Int. J. Obesity*, 18, 243, 1994.

90. Schwartz, R.S. et al., The effect of intensive endurance exercise training on body fat distribution in young and older men, *Metabolism*, 40, 545, 1991.

91. Andersson, B. et al., The effects of exercise training on body composition and metabolism in men and women, *Int. J. Obesity*, 15, 75, 1991.

92. Coon, P.J. et al., Effects of body composition and exercise capacity on glucose tolerance, insulin, and lipoprotein lipids in healthy older men: a cross-sectional and longitudinal intervention study, *Metabolism*, 38, 1201, 1989.

93. Poehlman, E.T. et al., Effects of resistance training and endurance training on insulin sensitivity in non-obese, young women: a controlled, randomized trial, *J. Clin. Endocrinol. Metab.*, 85, 2463, 2000.

94. DiPietro, L. et al., Moderate-intensity aerobic training improves glucose tolerance in aging independent of abdominal adiposity, *J. Am. Geriatr. Soc.*, 46, 875, 1998.

95. Treuth, M.S. et al., Reduction in intra-abdominal adipose tissue after strength training in older women, *J. Appl. Physiol.*, 78, 1425, 1995.

96. Bouchard, C. et al., The response to exercise with constant energy intake in identical twins, *Obesity Res.*, 2, 400, 1994.

97. Schwartz, R.S. et al., The effect of intensive endurance exercise training on body fat distribution in young and older men, *Metabolism*, 40, 545, 1991.

98. Després, J.-P. et al., Loss of abdominal fat and metabolic response to exercise training in obese women, *Am. J. Physiol. Endocrinol. Metab.*, 261, E159, 1991.

99. Després, J.-P. and Lamarche, B., Effects of diet and physical activity on adiposity and body fat distribution: implications for the prevention of cardiovascular disease, *Nutr. Res. Rev.*, 6, 137, 1993.

100. Williams, M.J. et al., Intra-abdominal adipose tissue cut-points related to elevated cardiovascular risk in women, *Int. J. Obesity*, 20, 613, 1996.

101. Ross, R. and Janssen, I., Is abdominal fat preferentially reduced in response to exercise-induced weight loss? *Med. Sci. Sports Exerc.*, 31, S568, 1998.

102. Ross, R., Freeman, J.A., and Janssen, I., Exercise alone is an effective strategy for reducing obesity and related co-morbidities, *Exerc. Sport Sci. Rev.*, 28, 165, 2000.

103. Ross, R., Janssen, I., and Tremblay, A., Obesity reduction through lifestyle modification, *Can. J. Appl. Physiol.*, 25, 1, 2000.

104. Ohlson, L.O. et al., The influence of body fat distribution on the incidence of diabetes mellitus, 13.5 years of follow-up of the participants of the study of men born in 1913, *Diabetes*, 34, 1055, 1985.

105. Kannel, W.B. et al., Regional obesity and risk of cardiovascular disease: the Framingham study, *J. Clin. Epidemiol.*, 44, 183, 1991.

106. Rexrode, R.M. et al., Abdominal adiposity and coronary heart disease in women, *JAMA*, 280, 1843, 1998.

107. Frayne, K.N., Visceral fat and insulin resistance: causative or correlative? *Br. J. Nutr.*, 83, S71, 2000.

108. Hill, J.O. et al., Racial differences in amounts of visceral adipose tissue in young adults: the CARDIA (Coronary Artery Risk Development in Young Adults) study, *Am. J. Clin. Nutr.*, 69, 381, 1999.

109. Conway, J.M. et al., Visceral adipose tissue differences in black and white women, *Am. J. Clin. Nutr.*, 61, 765, 1995.

*chapter eight*

# Effects of endurance exercise on total and regional adiposity in children

*Margarita S. Treuth*

## Contents

## 8.1   Introduction

Physical activity has been promoted as a lifelong positive health behavior in children and adolescents.[1] In adults, physical activity is associated with weight maintenance or weight loss. In children, it is more complicated because it is difficult to separate out the effects of the physical activity from normal growth and maturation.

Current data on physical activity levels in children are few. One study of over 4000 children from ages 8 to 16 showed that approximately 20% of U.S. children do not exercise vigorously more than twice per week, with the rate being higher in girls (26%) than in boys (17%).[2] The Centers for Disease Control and Prevention recommends that students in kindergarten to grade 12 (ages 5 to 18) have comprehensive, daily physical education; however, only 60% of high school students are enrolled in physical education classes, with only 25% taking daily physical education.[3]

Several studies have suggested that reduced physical activity plays a significant role in the etiology of childhood obesity.[4,5] In the Framingham Children's Study, preschool children with low levels of physical activity gained substantially more subcutaneous fat than did more active children.[6] In a 3-year longitudinal analysis of preschool children, increases in children's leisure activity and higher baseline aerobic activity were associated with decreases in body mass index.[7] This suggested that accelerated weight gain in preschool children could be modified by participation in physical activity.[7] In children followed from ages 5 to 9.5, a decrease in energy expenditure due to physical activity was observed in the girls, but not the boys.[8] A 50% reduction in physical activity was seen in this group of children, accompanied by an increase in fat mass. Insufficient levels of physical activity in children in the U.S. may lead to increases in adiposity. Promotion of physical activity in children should be a primary health goal.

## 8.2   Energy balance and physical activity

Physical activity is a key component of the energy balance equation. Energy balance is achieved when energy intake equals energy expenditure, and weight gain results when intake exceeds expenditure. Total energy expenditure (TEE) is comprised of basal/resting metabolic rate, the thermic effect of food, and activity energy expenditure (EE). Resting metabolic accounts for about 60 to 70% of the total energy expenditure; whereas, the thermic effect of food is much smaller (10%), and the activity component constitutes the remainder. Because resting metabolic rate accounts for a large portion of TEE, interindividual differences in the resting metabolic rate may contribute to the development of obesity. Individuals with a low resting metabolic rate are at risk for weight gain, whereas those with high activity EE are less likely to become overweight.

Mayer et al.[9,10] first suggested the existence of a threshold of inactivity that was associated with poor weight control. Persons with high levels of physical activity can maintain an energy balance, but those with low physical activity cannot regulate this balance as precisely; therefore, they become overweight. Physical activity level (PAL = TEE/resting metabolic rate) can be quantified using a highly accurate technique, namely doubly labeled water. From existing data sets of doubly labeled water, fat mass (FM), and fat-free mass (FFM), a higher PAL was associated with a lower fat mass in males.[11] Schulz and Schoeller[12] found a highly significant negative relationship between PAL and body fatness, suggesting that a low PAL is a permissive factor for obesity. The threshold of physical activity that protects against weight gain is 1.75, as supported by cross-sectional, doubly labeled water data in adults.[13] This threshold, however, has not been examined in children; furthermore, these issues are complicated by the fact that children also require energy for growth.

Several well-designed studies on children at risk of becoming obese by virtue of parental obesity have yielded conflicting results as to whether energy expenditure plays a role in the development of obesity. Roberts et al.[14] reported that total energy expenditure was lower in 18 infants with overweight mothers than those of underweight mothers, but these results were not substantiated by two recent studies of infants of obese mothers.[15,16] Griffiths and Payne[17] found that TEE determined by heart rate monitoring and resting EE were lower in 20 overweight 4- to 5-year-old children with one obese parent or with two normal-weight parents. Both studies indicated that the differences in TEE were partially accounted for by a lower activity EE. Wurmser et al.[18] reported that preadolescent girls with two obese parents had the lowest resting EE. In contrast, Goran et al.[19] reported no differences in TEE and activity EE measured by doubly labeled water in 73 normal weight and overweight boys and girls predisposed to obesity. Treuth et al.[20] designed a study to determine whether energy expenditure, measured by 24-hour calorimetry and doubly labeled water, differs among normal-weight-for-height, multi-ethnic, prepubertal girls. The children were grouped according to parental leanness or overweightness/obesity, as classified by body mass index (BMI). Basal metabolic rate, sleeping metabolic rate, 24-hour EE, and activity counts were similar among familial groups. No significant familial group differences in free-living TEE, activity EE, or physical activity level were observed. Thus, it appears that physical activity energy expenditure may play some role in the development of obesity in children, but the literature is not conclusive.

## 8.3    Physical activity levels in children

Several studies assessing energy expenditure and activity have been conducted in children, from the preschool-age years through adolescence, as measured by the doubly labeled water technique. A review by Torun et al.[21] indicated that the PAL has ranged from 1.38 to 1.51 in studies including children 2.5 to 5.5 years old. In 5-year-old white children, the energy cost of physical activity accounted for only $16 \pm 7\%$ of TEE (physical activity level = 1.37).[22] Another study in 5-year-olds found a PAL of 1.38, with activity EE ranging from −54 to 1621 kcal/day.[19] In both studies, low levels of activity were observed. In two studies of 3- to 4.5-year-old children,[23,24] PALs of 1.47 and 1.52 in boys and 1.46 and 1.52 in girls were reported. In a compilation of all studies to date in 1- to 6-year-old children using doubly labeled water, the TEE was approximately 20% below current international recommendations, suggesting that the reduction is probably due to changes in levels of physical activity.[24]

The review by Torun et al.[21] also included physical activity levels in older children. The range from several studies of PALs for boys 6 to 13 years of age was 1.71 to 1.86, with a mean of 1.79 ± 0.06. Correspondingly, for girls, the range was 1.69 to 1.90, with a mean of 1.80 ± 0.12. Treuth et al.[20] reported PALs in the free-living situation of prepubertal girls with different predispositions to obesity. A wide range of PALs was found in the entire group (1.1 to 2.48), indicating that some children were very sedentary and some highly active in the free-living situation. For adolescent children over the age of 14 years, the mean for boys was 1.84 ± 0.05 (range, 1.79 to 1.88); for girls, 1.69 ± 0.03 (range, 1.67 to 1.69).[21]

Thus, it appears that preschool children have lower physical activity levels, as measured by doubly labeled water, than prepubertal or adolescent children. However, the optimal physical activity level to prevent excessive weight gain in these different age groups of children is not clear. Longitudinal studies are needed to monitor physical activity levels and normal growth patterns.

## 8.4   Childhood intervention studies

Several excellent reviews on childhood physical activity, obesity, and interventions have been published.[25–27] Story[25] provides a summary of school-based obesity intervention treatment studies. Out of 11 interventions, only one did not include a physical activity component. Overall, the interventions produced positive, but modest, short-term results in terms of reductions in obesity. Resnicow and Robinson[27] compiled a review on school-based studies targeting reduction of cardiovascular disease risk factors. They found that the positive effects of the intervention were the lowest for adiposity (16%) compared to other risk factors such as smoking and fitness.

One reason to design intervention studies is that the incorporation of physical activity in youth may lead to more active adults. Indeed, data from a large sample of adult men and women have shown that activity levels in the primary school years have a strong long-term effect on the activity habits of adults.[28]

The majority of studies that have examined the effects of physical activity on adiposity in children actually use the term *physical activity* rather than *endurance exercise*. The programs typically involve aerobic types of activities but are often used in conjunction with other components, such as strengthening/muscular-type training, behavioral techniques, or diet therapy. Also, the methods of measuring adiposity range from simple weight and height measures to more sophisticated measures, such as isotope dilution or dual-energy X-ray absorptiometry (DXA). Regional adiposity measures most often include skinfold and circumference measures, with a few studies reporting DXA and magnetic resonance imaging (MRI).

In this chapter, the focus is on physical activity interventions and their effects on weight and body composition. The effects on both total and regional adiposity are reviewed together.

## 8.5  Physical activity interventions and total adiposity

Although the effects of exercise or physical activity on body composition have been a fruitful area of research in adults, fewer well-controlled physical activity intervention studies have been reported in children. Intervention studies have been conducted in children and adolescents in which the primary outcome may or may not have been adiposity; however, in many of these studies weight and body composition were assessed. These studies will be discussed, as they provide information on the effects of physical activity on body composition. Results from physical activity intervention studies are controversial, with some studies showing beneficial changes in body composition,[29–33] while others have shown no effects.[34–39]

Intervention studies that have targeted obese children and were designed to reduce or prevent further obesity have been conducted in school-based settings. Some studies suggest that these interventions can significantly reduce the prevalence of obesity.[40,41] However, one study that was less well-controlled and of a short duration (1 month) did not report any significant changes in body composition.[42] Some of these interventions will be reviewed in greater detail and are separated out by the ages of the participants.

### 8.5.1  Preschool children

Preschool children underwent a school-based exercise program designed to evaluate obesity indices.[33] Kindergarten children ($n = 292$) either participated in a morning walk plus aerobic dance session 3 times a week or a control condition for approximately 30 weeks. The exercise group had a significant decrease in the prevalence of obesity (defined as the 95th percentile for BMI), decreasing from 12.2 to 8.8% by the end of the program. BMI in the girls decreased by 0.28 units compared to the controls. This study provides evidence that very young children can be targeted for intervention studies.

### 8.5.2  Prepubertal/pubertal children

One of the most widely cited studies in this age-group was by Epstein et al.[30] It involved obese 8- to 12-year-old children (mean age, 10.1 years) who were randomized to treatment groups that targeted decreasing sedentary behaviors and increasing physical activity. Sixty-one families participated in the study. Decreases in percentage overweight were found after the intervention in the sedentary group (–19.9) and exercise group (–13.2) after 4 months. After 1 year, the sedentary group had the greater decrease in percentage overweight and a greater decrease in percent body fat (–4.7%)

vs. the control (–1.3%).[30] Thus, this study demonstrated that reducing sedentary behaviors was more effective in altering body fatness than exercise alone or in combination with reducing sedentary behaviors in obese children. Whether or not this same type of intervention would be effective in younger or older children remains to be determined.

Burke et al.[34] enrolled 800 11-year-olds into 10-week interventions that incorporated physical activity into a program for higher risk children. The intervention consisted of classroom sessions along with 20-min fitness sessions. A physical activity enrichment program was given to the higher risk children and included physical activity diaries. Following the program, no differences in weight were observed between the intervention and control schools for the girls. Body mass index increased in all groups, but a greater decrease in subscapular skinfolds was found in the girls, especially the higher risk girls ($p < 0.03$). This was not observed in the boys. The authors suggested that including physical activity for high-risk children can produce benefits that persist for at least 6 months after the intervention finishes, and they point to the need for long-term programs.

In a school-based intervention study, Stephens et al.[43] implemented a supplemental physical activity program for low-income, minority, urban, elementary-school children. During the 15-week program, the children ($n = 45$; mean age, 8.4 years) attended their regular physical education class one time a week, but they also participated in the classroom physical activity for an additional three sessions each week. The classroom activity constituted 5 min of warm-up, followed by 20 min of continuous aerobic exercise and then a cool-down. The control group gained significantly more weight than the intervention group. A significant reduction in the sum of skinfolds (triceps and calf) also occurred in the experimental group. Although this reduction was significant, it was only 1.4 cm and is not physiologically impressive.

In 18 elementary schools, a randomized, controlled field trial was designed which consisted of a knowledge and attitude program and an adaptation of the physical education program.[32] The children ($n = 422$) had at least two risk factors (low aerobic power and either high cholesterol or obesity). An aerobic activity program (jump rope, aerobic dance, etc.) was taught 3 times a week. Although the primary outcome was cholesterol, BMI and body fat (skinfolds) were assessed. The intervention produced a small reduction in body fat in the intervention group vs. the control group, but no differences were observed for BMI.

A 3-year controlled intervention study in 10-year old Dutch children was implemented to determine the influence of physical activity on plasma lipid and lipoprotein profiles.[39] The intervention was comprised of additional physical education classes and afternoon out-of-school sports activities. Growth in weight and height, including skinfold measures, was the same between the intervention and control girls, with the intervention boys growing somewhat more slowly. Incidentally, the lipids and apoprotein profile did not change with the intervention in the boys, but a slight increase in triglycerides was observed in the intervention girls. The authors speculate that the intensity of the exercise may have been too low.[39]

A 2-year intervention was implemented in a rural community that involved changing the school menus and the physical activity of the intervention schools.[44] The existing classroom teachers implemented the physical activity component, which consisted of aerobic activities for 30 to 40 min, 3 days a week. The children were 9.2 years of age at the start of the study and 10.7 years by completion. Absolute body fat decreased from baseline to the end of year 2 in the intervention group ($-2.5 \pm 5.9$ kg) and in the control group ($-2.7 \pm 6.9$ kg); however, in terms of percent body fat (%BF), both groups increased slightly. Thus, this type of intervention was unsuccessful in terms of reducing the relative amount of body fat in children.

The Sports, Play, and Active Recreation for Kids (SPARK) program was a school-based intervention with three components: a specialist-led condition, a teacher-led condition, and a control condition.[37,38] Seven elementary schools ($n = 955$) participated in the study. The primary outcome was physical activity, in which the children in the specialist-led group spent more time being physically active. Height, weight, and calf and triceps skinfolds were measured over 2 years. The data showed a nonsignificant trend for children exposed to specialized physical education to have lower total body fat after the 2 years.[38]

The Child and Adolescent Trial for Cardiovascular Health (CATCH) study was designed to improve physical activity in children grades 3 through 5.[45] The program involved both the schools and the parents at home in promoting physical activity. Physical activity was assessed by several methods, including self-report, direct observation, and a timed run test. The results showed that physical activity was increased in the intervention schools, as measured by direct observation and by self-report. As part of the CATCH cohort, Simons-Morton et al.[46] reported on the average activity levels in these elementary-school children. Body mass index was not associated with moderate to vigorous, vigorous, and sedentary activity in mixed models analyses of covariance.

## 8.5.3 Adolescence

A follow-up study of the children enrolled in the CATCH trial provided information regarding the physical activity and BMI at grade 8.[36] The children in the intervention schools maintained significantly higher physical activity levels than control children; however, no differences in BMI were found. Thus, the original CATCH study was successful in modifying physical activity and dietary behaviors, and these positive behaviors continued without further intervention;[36] however, the intervention did not significantly alter weight, height, or body composition.

## 8.6   Endurance exercise

### 8.6.1   Total/regional adiposity

A few studies have used short-term exercise training programs to evaluate the effects of exercise on obesity and other health risk factors. In an analysis of 71 obese children who underwent 4 months of physical training, the variables that explained 25% of the variance of the change in body fat with the training included age, vigorous activity, diet, and baseline percentage body fat.[47] Details on these training studies will be provided in this section, including the exercise prescription.

Obese boys were given an exercise program for 4 weeks that involved cycling at 50 to 60% of VO$_2$max for 45 min.[48] The ten boys, ages 10 to 11, did not significantly change their body fatness as measured by deuterium and [18]O dilution and densitometry (32.4 to 31.7%). This short-term exercise program did not alter body fatness, but did increase the free-living energy expenditure outside the training. This has important implications for energy balance, and it remains to be determined whether the same program would have altered total adiposity if the program were continued in these same children over a longer period of time.

Gutin et al.[31] enrolled obese, 7- to 11-year-old black girls in a supervised physical training program with no dietary restriction. A lifestyle intervention was also implemented in a matched sample of girls. The physical training consisted of five 40-min sessions each week for 10 weeks, at an intensity of at least 60% of maximal heart rate. The exercises included group aerobics, cycling, walking/jogging, circuit training, rope jumping, and cross-country ski machine. Body composition was measured by DXA. The percent fat of the physical training group decreased significantly by 1.4%, along with a slight reduction in fat mass. Fat-free mass increased in both groups. Regional body composition (FM and FFM) in the trunk and extremities was also examined. Fat-free mass of the extremities significantly increased (by 0.86 kg), whereas no significant changes were observed for the trunk. Fat mass did not change significantly in either region. Thus, this study demonstrated that a strict physical training program for obese, prepubertal, black girls was able to reduce total body fatness.[31]

One study specifically targeted the reduction of both total body fat and visceral fat.[49] Children 7 to 11 years of age participated in a 4-month physical training program (40 min/session, 5 days/week, heart rate of 157 bpm). Total body composition was measured by DXA, and visceral adipose tissue was measured by MRI. The results showed that the children in the intervention groups increased visceral adipose tissue significantly less than the control group.[49] The training group increased visceral adipose tissue by only 1.3 cm$^3$, compared to a 20.9-cm$^3$ increase in the controls. Subcutaneous adipose tissue decreased in the exercise group (–16.2 cm$^3$) and increased in the control (+48.9 cm$^3$). In terms of total body composition, total %BF (–2.2%) and FM (–0.8 kg) decreased, and FFM increased (+1.9 kg). Thus, this study demonstrated positive changes in body composition resulting from an aerobic exercise program (without dietary restriction) for obese children.

Another study by the same group[50] randomly assigned a group of children to physical training for 4 months and then assigned another group to complete the training program 4 months later. The children ($n$ = 79, 7 to 11 years of age) exercised 40 min/session, 5 days/week. Both groups reduced body fatness by 1.6% after the training, with the group who exercised the first 4 months regaining 1.3% fat by the end of the study.

Rowland and Boyajian[51] studied 24 girls and boys (10.9 to 12.8 years old) enrolled in an intervention designed to improve aerobic fitness. The children completed 30 min of aerobic activity 3 times a week for 12 weeks. The program replaced the usual physical education class in the school and consisted of running, aerobic dance, stair climbing, jumping rope, basketball, and other aerobic games. Weight and skinfolds (triceps and subscapular) were measured. Weight significantly increased after the aerobic training; however, no changes were observed in the sum of the two skinfolds. $VO_2max$ was improved with the training by 6.5%. Thus, this type of intervention did affect aerobic fitness but not body composition in children.

In conclusion, studies that are specifically designed with an aerobic exercise training protocol have shown mixed results as to whether or not physical activity can modify total or regional adiposity. Further studies are required in this area to define the effects of physical activity on body composition.

## 8.6.2    Diet effects on adiposity

The use of exercise combined with diet to reduce adiposity has been examined in children.[52-55] A review of this topic reported a reduction in body weight and fat in obese children of 5 to 20% after both a physical activity and a low-calorie diet program, ranging from 3 to 29 weeks in duration.[56] Generally, these studies reported a reduction in body weight or fatness.

In one study, obese children underwent a diet and endurance exercise program for 12 weeks.[52] Five children (8 to 10 years of age) reduced their energy intake by –500 to –600 kcal/day for the 12-week period. A walking program of 5 days per week was introduced for the last 6 weeks of the study. Only weight, not body composition, was assessed. The children lost a significant amount of weight on the program (4.2 ± 0.4 kg).

A 3-year exercise and diet intervention was tested in obese boys and girls ages 7 to 17.[55] A home-based moderate-intensity exercise (45 to 55% $VO_2max$) program was prescribed, which included aerobic, strength, and flexibility exercises. Supervised exercise sessions for 30 to 40 min were also incorporated at the medical center. After the initial 10-week intervention, the children lost an average of 9 kg, with a significant decrease in body fatness. By the end of the 3-year intervention, no further significant changes in weight, percent ideal body weight, or percent body fat were observed.

Epstein et al.[53] reported on a 10-year follow-up of obese children 6 to 12 years of age. The intervention consisted of a diet (traffic-light diet, with color coding of foods according to caloric density), aerobic exercise program (given information), and behavioral interventions. Children were divided into a child and parent group (reinforcing behavior change), a child group, and a control group. Follow-up at both 5 and 10 years showed significantly greater decreases in percent overweight of –11.2% and –7.5%, respectively, in the child-parent group compared with control. This was the first study to demonstrate long-term treatment effects of diet and exercise, combined with behavioral techniques, in obese children/adolescents.

### 8.6.3    Adiposity in special populations

Despite a lack of information on the effects of endurance exercise on special populations, studies have examined these effects in children with cerebral palsy[57] and insulin-dependent diabetes mellitus.[58]

The effects of a 9-month sports program on adiposity, fitness, and physical activity were examined in children with spastic cerebral palsy.[57] Twenty children (mean age, 9.2 years) and matched controls participated. The program consisted of either 2 or 4 sessions per week. The control group increased fat mass after the 9 months by 1.1 ± 1.6 kg, whereas the intervention group remained the same ($p < 0.05$). The conclusion was that aerobic training in children with cerebral palsy was beneficial in terms of aerobic power and maintenance of body composition, but it did not alter physical activity levels as measured by calorimetry.

A comparison was made between adolescent males with insulin-dependent diabetes mellitus and a control group to determine the effects of a training program on fitness, body composition, muscle strength, and glucose regulation.[58] Adolescent males ($n = 20$) underwent a mixed endurance and calisthenic/strength program 3 times a week for 12 weeks. Both groups reduced their %BF with the training program. The diabetic males also increased their FFM by 3.5%. The authors concluded that aerobic circuit training is safe for properly trained and monitored diabetic adolescents.

## 8.7    Future directions

Many school-based intervention studies have been conducted in prepubertal and pubertal children. What is lacking is the implementation of such programs in the very young (preschool age) as well as in middle-school and high-school children. The effects of physical activity intervention on body fatness in adolescent children are particularly important given the high rates of obesity in this age group. Also, sedentary activities (computers and television viewing) occupy a particularly great amount of time in these children. Targeting these behaviors along with physical activity would be desirable. It is also important to target very young (3- to 5-year-old) children, as incorporation/learning of an active lifestyle at an early age may be critically important for future health behaviors.

Little information is available on the long-terms effects of physical activity on body composition in children. It would be valuable to have a long-term follow-up on the children who have participated in the previously reviewed studies to determine whether the interventions had any long-lasting effects.

Another potential area of interest would be to determine the optimal training program to produce beneficial effects on body composition. The optimal frequency, intensity, and duration of physical activity to be implemented in programs for children are not clearly defined. This information would be highly valuable as researchers, health professionals, and school educators try to alter their implementation of these types of programs.

The influence of endurance exercise training on regional adiposity is limited. Use of sophisticated measures of regional adiposity is warranted to determine whether exercise influences visceral or intra-abdominal fat or subcutaneous abdominal fat.

## 8.8 Summary

The literature reflects a consensus that maintenance of body weight and composition is highly important in terms of health consequences for children; therefore, many different interventions have been implemented at clinical centers, in schools, and in homes. Different exercise prescriptions (intensities, durations, frequencies) have also been tried. Specific studies using aerobic exercise are, however, limited.

The effects of growth and maturation on the outcomes make it difficult to provide an overall finding. In addition, studies have used varied body composition measures, and it is not always easy to compare among the studies. Thus, the interpretation of the findings is influenced by the method used to measure adiposity, along with the type of program that was implemented. However, it appears that the general consensus is that physical activity can improve body composition to some degree.

## References

1. Kohl, H.W., Hobbs, K.E., Development of physical activity behaviors among children and adolescents, *Pediatrics*, 101, 549, 1998.
2. Andersen, R.E., Crespo, C.J., Bartlett, S.J., Cheskin, L.J., and Pratt, M., Relationship of physical activity and television watching with body weight and level of fatness among children, *JAMA*, 279, 938, 1998.
3. U.S. Department of Health and Human Services (USDHHS), Public Health Service, Centers for Disease Control and Prevention (CDC), Guidelines for school and community programs to promote lifelong physical activity among young people, *Morbid. Mortal. Wkly. Rev.*, 46, 1, 1997.
4. Berkowitz, R.I., Agras, W.S., Korner, A.F., Kraemer, H.C., and Zeanah, C.H., Physical activity and adiposity: a longitudinal study from birth to childhood, *J. Pediatr.*, 106, 734, 1985.

5. Eck, L.H., Klesges, R.C., Hanson, C.L., and Slawson, D., Children at familial risk for obesity: an examination of dietary intake, physical activity and weight status, *Int. J. Obesity*, 16, 71, 1992.

6. Moore, L.L., Nguyen, U.S., Rothman, K.J., Cupples, L.A., and Ellison, R.C., Preschool physical activity level and change in body fatness in young children. The Framingham Children's Study, *Am. J. Epidmiol.*, 142(9), 982, 1995.

7. Klesges, R.C., Klesges, L.M., Eck, L.H., and Shelton, M.L., A longitudinal analysis of accelerated weight gain in preschool children, *Pediatrics*, 95(1), 126, 1995.

8. Goran, M.I., Gower, B.A., Nagy, T.R., and Johnson, R.K., Developmental changes in energy expenditure and physical activity in children: evidence for a decline in physical activity in girls before puberty, *Pediatrics*, 101, 887, 1998.

9. Mayer, J., Marshall, J.J., Vitale, J.U., Christensen, J.H., Mashayki, M.B., and Stare, F.J., Exercise, food intake, and body weight in normal rats and genetically obese adult mice, *Am. J. Physiol.*, 177, 544, 1954.

10. Mayer, J., Roy, P., and Mitra, K.P., Relation between calorie intake, body weight and physical work: studies in an industrial male population in West Bengal, *Am. J. Clin. Nutr.*, 4, 169, 1956.

11. Westerterp, K.R., Alterations in energy balance with exercise, *Am. J. Clin. Nutr.*, 68, 970S, 1998.

12. Schulz, L.O., and Schoeller, D.A., Compilation of total daily energy expenditures and body weights in healthy adults, *Am. J. Clin. Nutr.*, 61, 4, 1995.

13. Schoeller, D.A., Balancing energy expenditure and body weight, *Am. J. Clin. Nutr.*, 68, 956S, 1998.

14. Roberts, S.B., Savage, J., Coward, W.A., Chew, B., and Lucas, A., Energy expenditure and energy intake in infants born to lean and overweight mothers, *N. Engl. J. Med.*, 318, 461, 1988.

15. Davies, P.S., Wells, J.C., Fieldhouse, C.A., Day, J.M., and Lucas, A., Parental body composition and infant energy expenditure, *Am. J. Clin. Nutr.*, 61, 1026, 1995.

16. Stunkard, A.J., Berkowitz, R.I., Stallings, V.A., and Schoeller, D.A, Energy intake, not energy output, is a determinant of body size in infants, *Am. J. Clin. Nutr.*, 69, 524, 1999.

17. Griffiths, M., and Payne, P.R., Energy expenditure in small children of obese and non-obese parents, *Nature*, 260, 698, 1976.

18. Wurmser, H., Laessle, R., Jacob, K., Langhard, S., Uhl, H., Angst, A., Muller, A. and Pirke, K.M., Resting metabolic rate in preadolescent girls at high risk of obesity, *Int. J. Obesity*, 22, 793, 1998.

19. Goran, M.I., Carpenter, W.H., McGloin, A., Johnson, R., Hardin, M.J., and Weinsier, R.L., Energy expenditure in children of lean and obese parents, *Am. J. Physiol.*, 268, E917, 1995.

20. Treuth, M.S., Butte, N.F., and Wong, W.W., Effects of familial predisposition to obesity on energy expenditure in multiethnic prepubertal girls, *Am. J. Clin. Nutr.*, 71, 893, 2000.

21. Torun, B., Davies, P.S.W., Livingstone, M.B.E., Paolisso, M., Sackett, R., and Spurr, G.B., Energy requirements and dietary recommendations for children and adolescents 1 to 18 years old, *Eur. J. Clin. Nutr.*, 50(1), S37, 1998.

22. Fontvielle, A.M., Harper, I.T., Ferraro, R.T., Spraul, M., and Ravussin, E., Daily energy expenditure by five-year-old children, measured by doubly labeled water, *J. Pediatr.*, 123, 200, 1993.

23. Davies, P.S.W., Livingstone, M.B.E., Prentice, A.M., Coward, W.A., Jagger, S.E., Stewart, C., Strain, J.J., and Whitehead, R.G., Total energy expenditure during childhood and adolescence, *Proc. Nutr. Soc.*, 50, 14A, 1991.
24. Davies, P.S.W., Total energy expenditure in young children, *Am. J. Hum. Biol.*, 8, 183, 1996.
25. Story, M., School-based approaches for preventing and treating obesity, *Int. J. Obesity*, 23(2), S43, 1999.
26. Goran, M.I., Figueroa, R., McGloin, A., Nguyen, V., Treuth, M.S., and Nagy, T.R., Obesity in children: recent advances in energy metabolism and body composition, *Obesity Res.*, 3, 277, 1995.
27. Resnicow, K., and Robinson, T.N., School-based cardiovascular disease prevention studies: review and synthesis, *Ann. Epidemiol.*, S7, S14, 1997.
28. Trudeau, F., Laurencelle, L., Tremblay, J., Rajic, M., and Shephard, R.J., Daily primary school physical education: effects on physical activity during adult life, *Med. Sci. Sports Exerc.*, 31(1), 111, 1999.
29. Bush, P., Zuckerman, A.E., Taggart, V.S., Theiss, P.K., Peleg, E.O., and Smith, S.A., Cardiovascualr risk factor prevention in black school children: the "Know Your Body" evaluation project, *Health Educ. Q.*, 16, 215, 1989.
30. Epstein, L.H., Valoski, A.M., Vara, L.S., McCurley, J., Wisniewski, M., Kalarchian, M.A., Klein, K.R., and Shrager, L.R., Effects of decreasing sedentary behavior and increasing activity on weight change in obese children, *Health Psych.*, 14(2), 109, 1995.
31. Gutin, B., Cucuzzo, N., Islam, S., Smith, C., Moffatt, R., and Pargman, D., Physical training improves body composition of black obese 7- to 11-year-old girls, *Obesity Res.*, 3, 305, 1995.
32. Harrell, J.S., Gansky, S.A., McMurray, R.G., Bangdiwala, S.I., Frauman, A.C., and Bradley, C.B., School-based interventions improve heart health in children with multiple cardiovascular disease risk factors, *Pediatrics*, 102, 371, 1998.
33. Mo-suwan, L., Pongprapai, S., Junjana, C., and Puetpaiboon, A., Effects of a controlled trial of a school-based exercise program on the obesity indexes of preschool children, *Am. J. Clin. Nutr.*, 68, 1006, 1998.
34. Burke, V., Milligan, R.A.K., Thompson, C., Taggart, A.C., Dunbar, D.L., Spencer, M.J., Medland, A., Gracey, M.P., Vandongen, R., and Beilin, L.J., A controlled trial of health promotion programs in 11-year-olds using physical activity "enrichment" for higher risk children, *J. Pediatr.*, 132, 840, 1998.
35. Killen, J.D., Telch, M.J., Robinson, F.N., Maccoby, N., Taylor, C.B., and Farquhar, J.W., Cardiovascular disease risk reduction for tenth graders: a multiple-factor, school-based approach, *JAMA*, 260, 1728, 1988.
36. Nader, P.R., Stone, E.J., Lytle, L.A., Perry, C.L., Osganian, S.K., Kelder, S., Webber, L.S., Elder, J.P., Montgomery, D., Feldman, H.A., Wu, M., Johnson, C., Parcel, G.S., and Luepker, R.V., Three-year maintenance of improved diet and physical activity: the CATCH cohort, *Arch. Pediatr. Adolesc. Med.*, 153, 695, 1999.
37. Sallis, J.F., McKenzie, T.L., Alcaraz, J.E., Kolody, B., Hovell, M.F., and Nader, P.R., Project SPARK: effects of physical education on adiposity in children, *Ann. N.Y. Acad. Sci.*, 699, 127, 1993.
38. Sallis, J.F., McKenzie, T.L., Alcaraz, J.E., Kolody, B., Faucette, N., and Hovell, M.F., The effects of a 2-year physical education program (SPARK) on physical activity and fitness in elementary school students, *Am. J. Public Health*, 87, 1328, 1997.

39. Zonderland, M.L., Erich, W.B.M., Kortlandt, W., and Erkelens, D.W., Additional physical education and plasma lipids and apoproteins: a 3-year intervention study, *Ped. Exerc. Sci.,* 128, 1994.

40. Resnicow, K., School-based obesity prevention, *Ann. N.Y. Acad. Sci.,* 699, 154, 1993.

41. Walter, H.J., Hofman, A., Vaughan, R.D., and Wynder, E.L., Modification of risk factors for coronary heart disease: five-year results of school-based intervention trial, *N. Engl. J. Med.,* 318, 1093, 1988.

42. Cohen, C.J., McMillan, C.S., and Samuelson, D.R., Long-term effects of a lifestyle modification exercise program on the fitness of sedentary, obese children, *J. Sports Med. Phys. Fitness,* 31, 183, 1991.

43. Stephens, M.B., and Wentz, S.W., Supplemental fitness activities and fitness in urban elementary school classrooms, *Family Med.,* 30(3), 220, 1998.

44. Donnelly, J.E., Jacobsen, D.J., Whatley, J.E., Hill, J.O., Swift, L.L., Cherrington, A., Polk, B., Tran, Z.V., and Reed, G., Nutrition and physical activity program to attenuate obesity and promote physical and metabolic fitness in elementary school children, *Obesity Res.,* 4, 229, 1996.

45. Luepker, R.V., Perry, C.L., McKinlay, S.M., Nader, P.R., Parcel, G.S., Stone, E.J., Webber, L.S., Elder, J.P., Feldman, H.A., Hohnson, C.C., Kelder, S.H., and Wu, M. (for the CATCH collaborative group), Outcome of a field trial to improve children's dietary patterns and physical activity: the Child and Adolescent Trial for Cardiovascular Health (CATCH), *JAMA,* 275, 768, 1996.

46. Simons-Morton, B.G., McKenzie, T.H., Stone, E., Mitchell, P., Osganian, V., Strikmiller, P.K., Ehlinger, S., Cribb, P., and Nader, P.R., Physical activity in a multiethnic population of third graders in four states, *Am. J. Public Health,* 87, 45, 1997.

47. Barbeau, P., Gutin, B., Litaker, M., Owens, S., Riggs, S., and Okuyama, T., Correlates of individual differences in body composition changes resulting from physical training in obese children, *Am. J. Clin. Nutr.,* 69(4), 705, 1999.

48. Blaak, E.E., Westerterp, K.R., Bar-Or, O., Wouters, L.J.M., and Saris, W.H.M., Total energy expenditure and spontaneous activity in relation to training in obese boys, *Am. J. Clin. Nutr.,* 55, 777, 1992.

49. Owens, S., Gutin, B., Allison, J., Riggs, S., Ferguson, M., Litaker, M., and Thompson, W., Effect of physical training on total and visceral fat in obese children, *Med. Sci. Sports Exerc.,* 31(1), 143, 1999.

50. Gutin, B., Owens, S., Okuyama, T., Riggs, S., Ferguson, M., and Litaker, M., Effect of physical training and its cessation on percent fat and bone density of children with obesity, *Obesity Res.,* 7(2), 208, 1999.

51. Rowland, T.W. and Boyajian, A., Aerobic response to endurance exercise training in children, *Pediatrics,* 96, 654, 1995.

52. Ebbeling, C.B. and Rodriquez, N.R., Effects of exercise combined with diet therapy on protein utilization in obese children, *Med. Sci. Sports Exerc.,* 31(3), 378, 1999.

53. Epstein, L.H., Valoski, A., Wing, R.R., McCurley, M.A., Ten-year follow-up of behavioral, family-based treatment for obese children, *JAMA,* 264, 2519, 1990.

54. Reybrouck, T., Vinckz, J., Van den Berghe, G., and Vanderschueren Lodeweyckx, M., Exercise therapy and hypocaloric diet in the treatment of obese children and adolescents, *Acta Paediatr. Scand.,* 79, 84, 1990.

55. Suskind, R.M., Sothern, M.S., Farris, R.P., vonAlmen, T.K., Schumacher, H., Carlisle, L., Vargas, A., Escobar, O., Loftin, M., Fuchs, G., Brown, R., and Udall, J.N., Recent advances in the treatment of childhood obesity, *Ann. N.Y. Acad. Sci.,* 181, 1995.
56. Bar-Or, O., *Pediatric Sports Medicine for the Practitioner,* Springer-Verlag, New York, 1983.
57. Van den Berg-Emons, R.J., Van Baak, M.A., Speth, L., and Saris, W.H., Physical training of school children with spastic cerebral palsy: effects on daily activity, fat mass and fitness, *Int. J. Rehabil. Res.,* 21(2), 179, 1994.
58. Mosher, P.E., Nash, M.S., Perry, A.C., LaPerriere, A.R., and Goldberg, R.B., Aerobic circuit exercise training: effect on adolescents with well-controlled, insulin-dependent diabetes mellitus, *Arch. Phys. Med. Rehabil.,* 79(6), 652, 1998.

# *Index*

## A